Insulin Pump

(For Paediatrics)

By Dr Tawfik Muammar

Contents

The aim of this book i
About the author ii
Acknowledgements iii
Dedication iv
Abbreviations v

1 Introduction 1
1.1 Why do we need insulin? 2
1.2 Managing diabetes via insulin pump 3
1.3 Benefits of insulin pump therapy 4
1.4 Types of insulin pump 8
1.5 Insulin pump basics 11
1.6 HbA1c and blood glucose monitoring 12

2 First steps towards pump therapy 16
2.1 Preparing for pump therapy 17
2.2 Basal rate calculation and setting 25
2.3 Insulin to carbohydrate ratio calculation 30
2.4 Correction dose calculation 32
2.5 Pump technical issues/failure 35
2.6 Removing the pump 35
2.7 Temporary basal rates 36
2.8 Keeping your emergency kit ready 36
2.9 Pump follow-up and support 36

3 Managing clinical issues of pump therapy 39
3.1 Managing pump therapy 40
3.2 Hypoglycaemia 40
3.3 Hyperglycaemia 46
3.4 Presence of ketones 50
3.5 Diabetic ketoacidosis (DKA) and illness 51
3.6 Testing and adjusting basal rate 52
3.7 Testing and adjusting insulin to carbohydrate ratio 56
3.8 Continuous glucose monitoring (CGM) 56
3.8 Meter/pump downloads, interpretation of blood glucose readings and decision making 68
3.9 Using CGM to manage difficult diabetes situations 74
3.10 Coming off the pump 75

4 Insulin pump and food 77
   4.1 Carbohydrate and glycaemic index 78
   4.2 Advanced bolus options 85

5 Life with an insulin pump 90
   5.1 School and social life 91
   5.2 Activity and exercise 92
   5.3 Illness 97
   5.4 Hospital admission for surgeries and severe illnesses 98
   5.5 Holidays and travel 100
   5.6 Ramadan and fasting 102
   5.7 Stressful and unplanned situations 103
   5.8 Puberty and menstruation 104
   5.9 Coffee and alcohol 105
   5.10 Steroids 105
   5.11 Psychological aspects of insulin pump therapy 106

6 Appendices 108
   Appendix I: Infection prevention 109
   Appendix II: Fasting record sheet 110
   Appendix III- Travel checklist 111
   Appendix IV: Management of hyperglycaemia in a patient on a pump 112
   Appendix V: Blood Glucose Conversion Chart (mmol/L - mg/dl) 112

The aim of this book

The aim of this book is to offer helpful information to healthcare professionals and parents to support children on insulin pump therapy. The book provides comprehensive information on a range of topics related to insulin pumps, including insulin action, diet, counting carbohydrates, pump use at school, exercise, use during illnesses, surgical operations and travelling with the pump.

This book is also designed to assist healthcare professionals, parents and children in the process of insulin pump initiation and to provide suggestions for the adjustment of basal and bolus insulin in all potential daily life situations. Reading this book with its clear information, tables and figures will help paediatric healthcare professionals, parents, carers and children get the most out of this valuable technology.

Every effort has been taken to ensure the information in this book is correct. However, it is the responsibility of the healthcare professionals to ensure they are happy with the information in the book and that the information given to children and parents is correct and in line with your local guidelines.

About the author

Dr Tawfik Muammar
MBBCh, DCH (UK), MRCPCH, MSc Diabetes (UK), CCT (UK)

Dr Muammar is a consultant paediatric diabetologist and endocrinologist at Imperial College London Diabetes Centre, Abu Dhabi. He has a strong clinical interest in paediatric diabetes and its related technology.

His interest began in 1996, when diabetes technology was not as advanced as it is now. Dr Muammar worked in North Africa initially, then consolidated his experience in the UK for more than a decade and currently works in the Middle East. His exposure to different environments and working with many experts has improved his way of thinking towards improving the care provided to children with diabetes.

Acknowledgments

I would like to acknowledge Dr Muna Al-Hasaeri, for her valuable scientific advice and comments.
I would also like to thank the following colleagues, who kindly reviewed this book:

Endocrinologists with special interest in diabetes technology
Dr Alero Adjene, MBBS, MRCP
Dr Ahmed Elaboudi, MBBS, MRCP (UK), PhD (UK)

Diabetes Specialist Nurse
Manar Abu Asaba

Clinical psychologist
Dr Sawsan Halawi, MSc (USA), PhD (USA)

Senior Dietician
Reem Khoury

Dedication

To Abdalmohiman, Taha and Yaken.

Abbreviations

BG	Blood glucose
BK	Blood ketone
BGL	Blood glucose level
CGM	Continuous glucose monitoring
CHO	Carbohydrate
CSII	Constant subcutaneous insulin infusion
DKA	Diabetic ketoacidosis
GI	Glycaemic index
h	Hour
HBA1c	Glycosylated haemoglobin A1c
Hypo	Hypoglycaemia
ICR	Insulin-to-carbohydrate ratio
IOB	Insulin on board
ISF	Insulin sensitivity factor
IV	Intravenous
MDI	Multiple daily injections
MARD	Mean absolute relative difference
NBM	Nil by mouth
Pre-op	Preoperative
TDDi	Total daily dose of insulin

1 Introduction

1.1 Why do we need insulin?
1.2 Managing diabetes via insulin pump
1.3 Benefits of insulin pump therapy
1.4 Types of insulin pump
1.5 Insulin pump basics
1.6 HbA1c and blood glucose monitoring

1.1 Why do we need insulin?

Our pancreas continually produces a small (background) amount of insulin. This background insulin is necessary to maintain blood glucose levels at night and between meals, whether we are eating or not. When food containing carbohydrate (CHO) is eaten, the pancreas produces exactly the appropriate amount of insulin to keep blood glucose levels within the normal range. The pancreas automatically decreases or increases insulin secretion according to changes in blood glucose level.

Figure 1.1 shows what happens in a child without diabetes. The peaks show the insulin that is secreted after breakfast, lunch and dinner. The height and shape of the peaks are determined by the amount and type of CHO eaten.

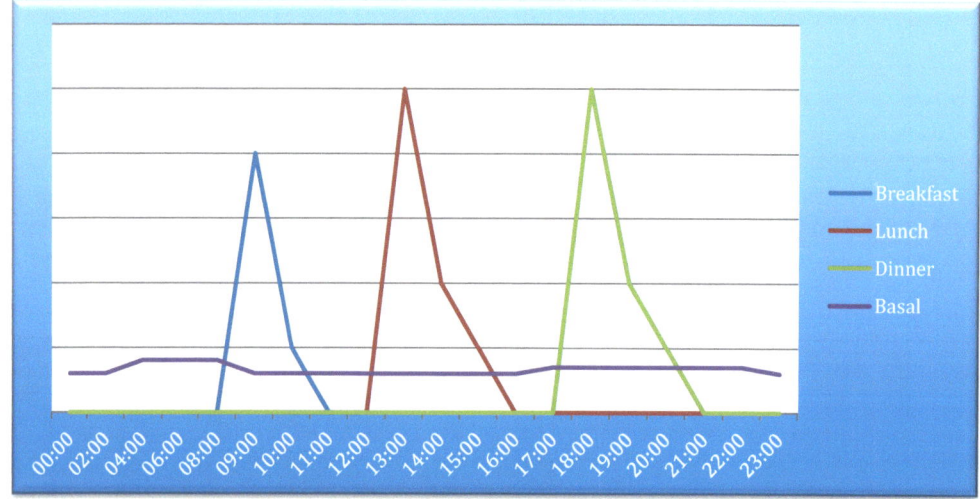

Figure 1.1 Insulin secretion in a child without diabetes

Diabetes results from an absolute or relative lack of the hormone insulin, leading to a high blood glucose concentration. In type 1 diabetes, an absolute deficiency of insulin occurs due to autoimmune destruction of the beta cells of the islets of Langerhans in the pancreas, which produce insulin. Children with type 1 diabetes require insulin treatment that may be delivered by a regimen of multiple daily injections (MDI) or insulin pump therapy (also known as 'continuous subcutaneous insulin infusion' or CSII).

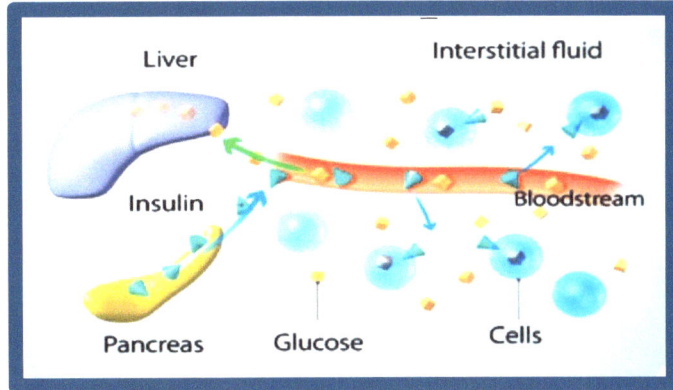

Figure 1.2 Insulin moves glucose into the cells and signals the liver to store any extra glucose that may be available and hence lowers BG level.

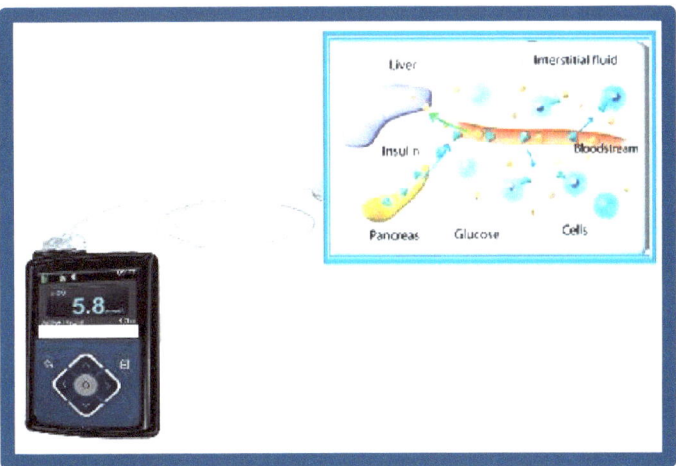

Figure 1.3 Infusion set and reservoir connects insulin pump and user.

1.2 Managing diabetes via insulin pump

Insulin pumps consist of a computerized syringe or pump and an infusion set, consisting of tubing and cannula. Insulin is held in a reservoir and is infused via an infusion set consisting of a flexible plastic tube (tubing) inserted into the subcutaneous tissue via a cannula (Figure 1.4).

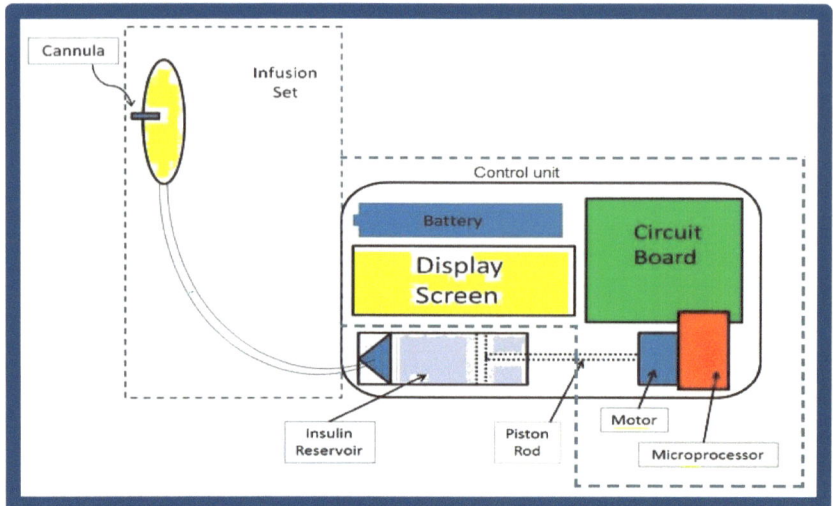

Figure 1.4 Insulin pump structure

Daily insulin requirements vary from child to child. The aim of insulin pump therapy is to mimic the pancreas; therefore, it delivers fast-acting insulin in two ways:
1- Background amount – called a 'basal rate'.
2- In response to food eaten or high blood glucose concentrations immediately or over a specified period of time – called a 'bolus'.

The pump delivers insulin in tiny amounts (microboluses), every few minutes over 24 hours, hence the term 'continuous subcutaneous insulin infusion' (CSII). Only fast-acting insulin is used in a pump. This means the patient doesn't need to eat extra meals or snacks, provided the basal rate is correct throughout the day. It is possible to have a different basal pattern set for those who are very active with sport (see exercise and activity section), during menstrual cycles (see section 5.8), or when blood glucose levels are high due to illness.

However, because only fast-acting insulin is used in the pump (i.e.no long-acting background insulin), action should be taken immediately if things go wrong with the insulin delivery.

The insulin commonly used is lispro (Humalog) or aspart (NovoRapid). In addition, a button can be pressed to deliver a bolus dose of insulin to cover CHO in the food eaten (food bolus) or give extra insulin to correct a high blood glucose level (correction bolus).

1.3 Benefits of insulin pump therapy

When considering why and when pumps should be used instead of injections, it is important to understand the differences between injections and pumps.

Variations in basal insulin requirements over a 24 hour period are common. Pumps have the ability to deliver small amounts of insulin over a planned period of time. This can be pre-programmed without the need to insert a needle every time. This means the insulin action can match closely and conveniently a child's insulin requirements.

The advantages and disadvantages of pumps over MDI are summarized in Table 1.1.
People often have reduced insulin requirements during sleep, with increasing requirement on waking. The insulin pump basal infusion rate can be programmed to fit that pattern in an individualized way. Similarly, basal rates can be reduced or discontinued with a pump at times of activity when insulin requirements are much lower. In contrast with MDI regimens, where rapid acting insulin can only be delivered once before the meal, insulin pumps allow for mealtime boluses to be delivered over a prolonged period of time (dual/extended bolus), enabling the insulin action to match the absorption of foods with low glycaemic index.

Pumps can also deliver very small volumes of insulin with finer control over changes in insulin delivery. Insulin pen devices and syringes can typically deliver insulin in increments of 0.5–1 unit, whereas pump increments are as low as 0.01–0.05 units. This is particularly useful for the insulin-sensitive and very young people with diabetes.

Table 1.1 Advantages and disadvantages of pumps

A-Advantages of pumps	B-Disadvantages
1- No need to inject every time insulin delivery is required. 2- Technology can motivate and improve engagement and self-management in children. 3-.Insulin delivery can be conveniently varied, allowing more flexibility.	1- No long-acting insulin, which increases the risk of rapid diabetic ketoacidosis (DKA) development if technical failure or interruption in insulin delivery. 2-Requires clinical support systems in place. 3- Constant attachment to pump. (Must be worn all the time, including when asleep).

4-Allows pre-programming of insulin to deliver variable amounts of insulin without constant input (e.g. while asleep or at school).	4-Pumps can only be disconnected for short periods (e.g. swimming).
5-Basal rates can be programmed to match activity, school physical education and changing requirements (e.g. puberty hormonal changes, menstrual periods, growth spurts, illness, travelling).	5-Set up for set changes is more complicated than for injections.
	6-Infusion sets and cannulas need to be changed every 2–3 days.
	7-Infusion site problems.
6- Reduces variations in insulin absorption.	8-Improper priming, air bubbles, tubing breaks and cannula kinks or dislodgment can interrupt insulin delivery and lead to DKA.
7- Bolus can be delivered over a varied time (e.g. slow absorption food and malabsorption conditions).	9-Infusion set problems.
	10-Risk of skin infections.
8-Deliver small doses (0.05–0.1 unit) versus 0.5–1 unit in a syringe/pen (useful for insulin-sensitive and very young children).	11-Requires a higher level of education, understanding and motivation for the best use of the pump to avoid and minimise problems.
9-Less insulin requirement.	More training required for patients and their families
10-Fewer snacks required.	
11-Tailored insulin delivery and reductions during hypoglycaemia and activity reduce the need for snacking.	12-More consultation slot time required.
12-Better integration with technology.	13-Pump costs, as well as running costs (accessories), are significantly higher than standard injections.
13-Temporary suspension or reduction of insulin delivery (example: during activity and in hypoglycaemia situations).	14-Increased healthcare provider training
	15-Constant visibility and reminder of diabetes.
14-Improved patient experience and satisfaction	16-Can affect perceived body image.

Limitations of pumps

Apart from closed-loop insulin delivery systems (sometimes called an 'artificial pancreas'), insulin pumps do not automatically adjust insulin delivery. Even sensor-augmented pumps require blood glucose testing and manual adjustment of the pump to match insulin delivery to requirements.

Pumps do not deliver insulin directly into the bloodstream and are dependent on the time taken for rapid-acting insulin to be absorbed from subcutaneous tissue (typically 15–20 min). They are also dependent on the amount of insulin on board. This means that even if a pump stops delivering insulin, insulin action may continue for some time. Even for rapid-acting analogue insulin, this is around 4 h - longer in specific situations - and varies from individual to individual.

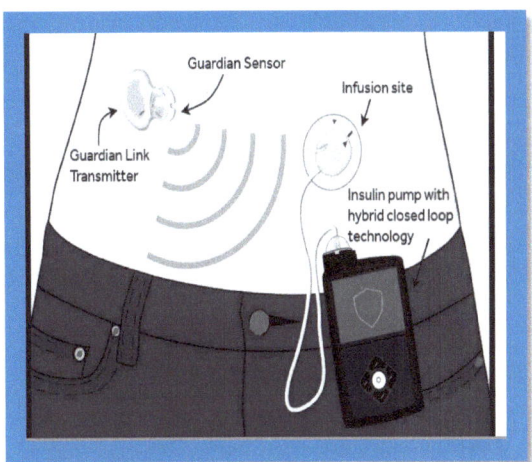

Figure 1.5 Sensor augmented pump

Insulin pumps (current evidence)

Meta-analysis of randomized controlled trials comparing insulin pumps with MDI in patients with type 1 diabetes have shown that insulin pump use resulted in better glycaemic control and is likely to reduce long-term diabetes complications, reduced frequency and severity of hypoglycaemia.

It also showed reduced glycaemic variability, which may be associated with oxidative stress and endothelial dysfunction.

Pump therapy also showed improved glycaemic control (HbA_{1c}) which is more dramatic for a higher baseline HbA_{1c}.

Moreover, RCTs showed reduced insulin requirements, improved patient performance and quality of life via providing flexibility in lifestyle and confidence-building.

Other uses of insulin pump therapy

Insulin pump therapy is considered to be safe and may be a valuable treatment for people with insulin-treated type 2 diabetes, and preliminary data suggest that HbA_{1c} improves with pump therapy. Current guidelines (which also incorporate cost–benefit estimates) do not advocate the routine use of pumps for type 2 diabetes.

The current evidence suggests benefits of insulin pump therapy for diabetes secondary to pancreatitis, pancreatic surgery-related diabetes and cystic fibrosis-related diabetes.

Barriers to pump therapy

Despite the clear evidence supporting pump therapy in type 1 diabetes, there are still some barriers to its widespread use:
1- Pump therapy should be offered to those who will clinically benefit from it and who can make use of it. Offering pumps to people where it may not be used appropriately, or where it may cause harm, must be avoided.
2- The cost of pumps, set-up and training makes pumps, consumables, accessories and replacements more expensive than injections.
3- Insulin pump therapy should be supported by a trained multidisciplinary pump team specializing in pump therapy (including a doctor, diabetes specialist nurse, dietician and access to a psychologist), who can provide structured education, with carbohydrate counting courses and advice on diet, exercise and lifestyle suitable for type 1 diabetes.

Pump choices

Insulin pumps vary in their size, features, complexity, simplicity, interface and colour. However, their unifying feature is the ability to programme and deliver small doses of insulin over a planned time.

1.4 Types of insulin pump

The two main types of insulin pump (tethered and patch pumps) are described in Table 1.2.

Table 1.2 Tethered and patch pumps

Pump type	Tethered pump	Patch pump (Figure 6)

Description	This is the most commonly used pump option. A long fine tube connects the pump to the cannula. The pump is then worn and may be visible. The pump is controlled by buttons on the pump itself or via a handheld device.	A more recent design. More discreet. Integrated standard cannula (no variation possible). A very short tube and cannula, which is integrated into a micro-pump device that attaches directly to the child's skin. The pump is controlled via a handheld device only.
Advantages	Some users prefer a tethered pump because of other features, such as continuous glucose sensing and the ability to place the pump in different places without moving the cannula (e.g. on a belt, in a pocket and under the pillow). One device for some pumps. Difficult to lose.	Patch pumps are popular due to their tubing-free design. Small size with minimal tubing. Good for infants and toddlers, it can be hidden under clothes. Difficult to remove by small children. Remote-controlled through handheld device and you don't need to disturb the child. Patch pumps are controlled via a handheld remote-control device. This wireless option is appealing to some and allows integration with capillary blood glucose meters. Lower risk of tube breakages or damage with patch pumps. Set changing is easier to perform with patch pumps with fewer steps involved.
Disadvantages	Tubing issues: kinks, dislodging and air bubbles.	If the remote is lost or malfunctions, pump control may be very limited. Two-piece device. More difficult to visualize the cannula insertion point or monitor and remove air bubbles manually. Currently, patch pumps do not have a CGM sensor link feature, but this may change in the future.

Patch pump

The handheld control device and patch micro-pump are shown below.

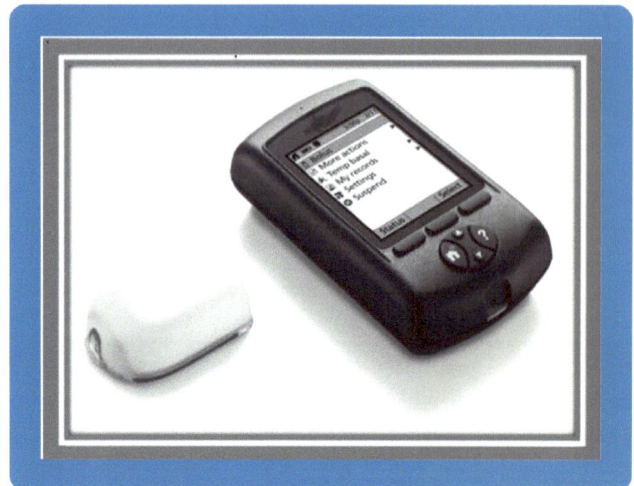

Figure 1.6 Patch pump and control device

How to choose between tethered and patch pumps

Table 1.2 summarized the differences between tethered pumps and patch pumps.

Although CSII is usually very successful, it is important that the benefits continue in the long term. The potential benefits include less frequent severe hypoglycaemia, return of early warning symptoms of hypoglycaemia, improved glucose control with less variability and better quality of life.

It would be expected that your patients would get a reduction in their HbA1c level of at least 0.25-0.5% less than their average level before starting on the pump (unless their HbA1c is less than 7.5% already).

To benefit from the pump, patients should be confident in using the technical features of the device. They should also be confident in measuring blood glucose levels, calculating correction doses and altering the amount of insulin depending on the CHO content of meals, activity or during illness.

We anticipate that you will see the benefits to your patient after 3-6 months of using the pump. These should be maintained in the longer term. It will be necessary to measure the benefits by checking your patient's HbA1c level, their hypoglycaemia awareness, and by gauging their quality of life (this may involve using questionnaires) at regular intervals.

1.5 Insulin pump basics

You need to teach your patients the basic functions of the pump (referring to the pump manufacturer's instruction booklet). This needs to cover both operational and clinical aspects such as:
- Inserting batteries
- Switching pump on/off
- Setting time and date
- How to fill up a cartridge/reservoir
- How to insert a cartridge
- Different infusion sets and insertion devices
- How to give a bolus
- How to set basal rates

Cannula sites

Figure 1.7 below shows the best sites in which to insert the cannula. It is advised to move within one area before changing to another completely.

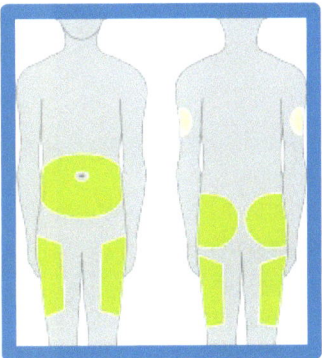

Figure 1.7 Cannula insertion sites

Cannula site management

1- Change infusion sets and reservoir every 2-3 days.
2- Avoid lumpy sites (lipohypertrophy) and heavily-used areas.
3- Infusion set should not be sited under the waistband or directly on the beltline. Also consider things like school/shoulder bags and seat belts.
4- Ensure cannula site rotation. The new infusion set should be inserted at least 3-5 cm away from the old site and 3cm away from umbilicus.
5- Applying local anaesthetic cream (EMLA or Ametop) to the skin prior to insertion is helpful for some children. Some children prefer to stand while inserting.

6- Do not remove the old infusion set until the new one is up and running. You may leave it in for up to 2 hours after insertion of the new one.
7- Do not forget to check for air bubbles in the tube – if present, remove the bubbles, these may considerably reduce the amount of insulin your patient is receiving.
8- Hold tube vertically when priming.
9- Avoid changing site late at night as you need to ensure that the cannula is working before the child goes to sleep, the best time to change site is about 30 minutes after a bath or before a meal, so that the food bolus ensures clearing of any tissue or blood left in the cannula.
10- Be aware that failure to absorb insulin overnight may result in ketones; therefore, avoid set changing before bedtime.
11- Disconnecting the pump from your patient's body is essential when priming, to avoid giving insulin unintentionally.
12- If you see blood in tubing, probably the cannula is sited in one of the small vessels and the infusion site should to be changed.
13- A slight stinging sensation may be experienced at the infusion sites after insertion. However if still painful after one hour it is best to change the site.
14- Check blood glucose level 2 hours after cannula insertion to ensure it is working.
15- Parents should inspect the cannula after removal to check for bending, kinks or signs of infection.

Suggested helpful points:
1- If infusion sets do not stick very well, consider an adhesive spray like Cavilon or wipes such as SkinPrep or Skin Tac that help with adhesion.
2- Remember that sweat, body heat, moisture, friction and hair may affect the infusion set tape as well. Check your infusion site and tape carefully.
3- Choose a site that will not be flexed or irritated during exercise.
4- Wear the pump away from the infusion site to avoid rubbing and friction.
5- If infusion sets are difficult or uncomfortable to remove, consider an adhesive remover such as Lift Plus.
6- Calendula or tea tree cream helps heal scars.
7- To prevent infection:
   a) Use a 'no touch' technique for ends of tubes.
   b) Wash hands before opening any package and after touching the old site.
   c) Change set if you suspect infection (pain, redness or discomfort).
   d) See Appendix I.

1.6 HbA1c and blood glucose monitoring

By regular blood glucose monitoring we can learn how different factors can affect the results, such as exercise, illnesses, food type, activities and stress. A patient's response to all of the above should help you know what's working and what to consider changing.

Average blood glucose testing, five times a day is necessary to achieve good results, and more often when aiming to improve control.

Table 1.3 Targets for glucose levels and HbA1c

Before each meal	90-140mg/dl (5-8 mmol/l)
Two hours after each meal	90-180mg/dl (5-10 mmol/l)
At night	80-160 mg/dl (4.5-9 mmol/l)
HbA1c	less than 58 mmol/mol (less than 7.5%)

Frequently asked questions from children/parents/carers:

1- **Why pump and not MDI?** See table 1.1 for advantages of the pump.
2- **Will my diabetes control improve?** It is easier to match your insulin to your blood glucose values.
3- **Where do I wear the pump?** You may prefer to wear it in your pocket or under your clothes. However, a variety of cases and accessories are available from the manufacturer and there are a number of organisations who also manufacture accessories.
4- **Can I ever take the pump off?** For better outcome the pump should be attached to your child almost constantly. However, the pump easily disconnects and you can take it off for about 1-2 hours for swimming, showering and exercise (contact sports). If you want to take it off for a longer time, you will need to take insulin injections during the time the pump is off.
5- **Will my child gain weight on the pump?** With better diabetes control, there is a tendency to gain weight. However, greater flexibility in timing of meals and food choices with the pump allows your child to manage weight more easily than on injection therapy.
6- **How do I learn to use the pump?** A certified pump trainer will teach them the pump's technical aspects and provide them with all the diabetes self-management skills necessary to use it. Most of the pump manufacturers have a 24-hour pump helpline for you to use whenever they have a question.

7- **What should I do if I shower?** Although most new pumps are waterproof, it is advised to disconnect the pump from the infusion set and re-insert after showering. The same applies for sauna and steam rooms. (Remember hot temperatures can accelerate insulin absorption.)
8- **What will happen to my pump during sleep?** Pumps can be kept strapped or clipped. Some children prefer having them under the pillow. Tubing should be long enough to allow this.
9- **Will the tube, cannula or pump compress if I roll over during sleep?** Cannulas do not compress but sleeping on them can be uncomfortable. Tubes are extremely durable and do not compress with normal daily use or during sleep.
10- **What should I do if swimming?** For prolonged periods over 4 hours, periodic bolus doses may be used or revert to multiple dose insulin injection regimen.
11- **Do I need any precautions when going through airport security X-rays?** Most pumps are safe to wear when going through security X-rays. However, it is best to check this with the device manufacturer. (If in doubt, remove.) For strong energy fields, such as CT scans or medical X-rays, it is advisable to disconnect from the insulin pump. Steel cannulas can be left in place.
12- **Do I need any special precautions during MRI scans?** Electrical device including pumps should not be exposed to strong electromagnetic fields, as it may damage them. Therefore, they must be disconnected and left outside the scanner room. Metal cannula must be removed.

Parents/children goals and expectations

Many people are initially resistant to pump therapy for reasons such as body image or feeling that the pump will be a constant reminder of diabetes. This can be resolved through discussion or meeting other pump users. Therefore, the healthcare team needs to ensure that patient/parent goals and expectations are reasonable and achievable.
The table below shows examples of realistic and unrealistic goals and expectations.

Table 1.5

Some realistic goals and expectations	Some unrealistic goals and expectations
1- To have better glucose control.	I don't want to check my blood sugar more than 3 times a day.
2- To avoid having frequent or severe hypoglycaemia, especially at night.	I don't want to give myself insulin shots ever again.

3- To add flexibility to lifestyle and eating habits.	I don't want to worry about diabetes.
4- To be able to sleep without worrying that my child has hypoglycaemia.	I don't want to carry diabetes supplies everywhere.
5- To be able to exercise without blood glucose going too low or too high.	

2 First steps towards pump therapy

2.1 Preparing for pump therapy
2.2 Basal rate calculation and setting
2.3 Insulin to carbohydrate ratio calculation
2.4 Correction dose calculation
2.5 Pump technical issues/ failure
2.6 Removing the pump
2.7 Temporary basal rates
2.8 Keeping your emergency kit ready
2.9 Pump follow-up and support

2.1 Preparing for pump therapy

Managing a patient on an insulin pump requires the same basic skills as managing a patient on multiple injection therapy. However, since the insulin pump separates the insulin used as background, or basal insulin, from the insulin needed for meal and corrections boluses, insulin can be matched to the metabolic need.

Before you start

Pre-pump, we need to select the right user, pump and cannula. Selecting the right user is the key for successful pump therapy. Consider your local clinical guidelines, indications and criteria for insulin pump therapy. You also need to take into account available evidence and cost effectiveness.

Before starting with insulin pump therapy, ensure that you have the pump, fast-acting insulin in a 10 ml vial, a reservoir/cartridge, the chosen cannula, infusion set, blood glucose monitor, ketone monitor, hypoglycaemia (hypo) remedy and a record of the total daily doses over the last week.

Indications

Pump therapy may be considered for children:
1- When MDIs are impractical or inappropriate.
2- When a patient has disabling (repeated and unpredictable) hypoglycaemia when attempting to reach target HbA_{1c} with MDIs, resulting in persistent anxiety about recurrence and an adverse effect on quality of life.
3- When a patient is unable to achieve a target HbA_{1c} of 7.5% or 58 mmol/mol with MDIs, including long-acting insulin analogues, despite a high level of care.

Selection criteria:

1- Patients and parents need to have realistic expectations of CSII and healthcare professionals need to ensure that patient/parent goals and expectations are reasonable and achievable (see Table 1.5).
2- Strong parental motivation.
3- Capacity to understand and use the pump. Parents need to be educated on the insulin pump to learn the basics of dealing with insulin pump and safety. It may not be an easy task for children or parents with learning difficulties or mental health issues.
4- Use carbohydrate counting, making insulin dosing adjustments appropriately with food and to correct blood glucose. Patient/parents need to know how to deal with daily changes and able to perform required pump adjustments

5- Perform/continue to perform self-monitoring of blood glucose (at least 4-5 times per day).
6- Understand the risks of insulin pump therapy.
7- Regularly engage with health services and professionals.
8- You may need an agreement of pump therapy between parents and the team.

What your patients need to know:

It is essential for your patients to have a basic understanding of diabetes management and to be comfortable with the mechanics of the pump before they start pumping. Even if they have had diabetes for many years, they should learn some new information before they begin pump therapy, including:

1- Theory of basal/bolus insulin therapy
2- Insulin action: onset, peak and duration
3- Carbohydrate counting
4- Self-monitoring blood glucose: how often and when
5- What causes low BG and how to treat it
6- What causes high BG and how to treat it
7- Ketones: what they are and when to check for them
8- Managing BG for sick days
9- Managing BG for changes in activity
10- Detailed record keeping
11- Inserting an infusion set
12- Programming/using their insulin pump

The education and support of children and parents working towards insulin pump therapy is the key to a successful outcome, this should include structured education for insulin dose adjustment and CHO counting.

Patients with type 1 diabetes must be able to count carbohydrates, manage activity and illness and be able to alter insulin in response to their blood glucose trends. This can be delivered via a structured carbohydrate counting course and other education programmes such as interactive training and support. On rare occasions, initiation of insulin pump therapy is clinically urgent and the requirement for education may be less important.

Selecting the pump

Pump selection depends on local availability; however, healthcare professionals should take into account the points in Table 2.1.

Table 2.1 Selecting the right pump

1-Healthcare professional experience	Pump therapy requires education and continuous support; therefore, healthcare professional experience is essential to support the long-term goals.
2- Choice and individual preference	Individual choices are important to get the best results because they are the ones who will be wearing and using the pump.
3- Consumables and technical support	Availability of technical support is an important consideration.
4-Other features	Depends on user requirements, such as being waterproof or ability to link with a continuous glucose sensor (sensor-augmented pump therapy).

Pump accessories

1- Cannulas:

Cannulas are available as steel and soft cannulas, can be inserted with an inserter or manually and are angled at 90° or 45°. Advantages and disadvantages of soft and steel cannulas are summarized in Table 2.2.

Table 2.2 Advantages and disadvantages of soft and steel cannulas

Type and description	Disadvantage	Advantage
Soft cannula is a flexible plastic material, made of Teflon. Introduced under the skin via a metal needle, which is removed, leaving the plastic cannula in the skin.	May kink or be bent under the skin, which can slow insulin delivery.	Is more comfortable. Recommended for children with nickel allergies.

Steel cannula Is hard and made of metal	Change every 48 hour (rather than 72 hours). Less comfortable.	Easy to insert. Bend and kink less. Useful in situations where reliability is desired due to lower risk of cannula slipping out or bending.

The point of skin entry of the cannula needle can be at 90° (perpendicular) to the skin or angled 20-45°.

Table 2.3 The advantages and disadvantages of angled and 90° cannula insertion

	Angled (20-45°) Longer cannula inserted at an angle.	90° (Shorter cannula inserted perpendicular to the skin)
Advantages	Better for leaner person. Less prone to falling out and kinking. Parents can see whether the catheter is inserted in the skin (it has a window at the insertion point in the adhesive dressing).	Less visibility of the needle Good for needle phobic children. Useful for insertion in arms, buttocks or hips (difficult to reach sites). Often done with insertion device.
Disadvantages	Harder to insert if there are visual or manual dexterity problems and in difficult-to-reach areas.	Risk of inserting into muscle in lean children. Less visibility of needle to confirm successful insertion.

Tubing and cannula length

The tubing length is usually influenced by a child's height, changing clothes, exercising, using the washroom, where they choose to wear the pump and placement of the pump while sleeping. Tubing lengths ranges between 45 and 107 cm.

Cannulas come in different lengths. The 90° cannulas are 6-13 mm in length, while angled cannulas are up to 12 mm long. Longer length cannulas have less risk of slippage but an increased risk of being inserted into muscle. Longer cannulas are recommended in obese children, frequent issues with cannula slippage, higher insulin requirements (≥25 unit boluses or ≥2.5 units/h basal) or lipohypertrophy.

The gauge of the needle refers to its thickness (with smaller gauges being thicker). Larger gauges may be more suited to people with a higher BMI or where there may be a risk of kinking or bending. Usual sizes are between 25 gauge and 29 gauge.

Tube disconnection

Children may need to disconnect themselves from the pump and tubing, while leaving the cannula inserted (e.g. swimming, showering and exercise). To facilitate this, there are various disconnection mechanisms. The two main types are 'sideways pull disconnection' mechanisms and 'twist and lift off'. The latter is easier to disconnect, but harder to reconnect in difficult-to-access areas. The former has a 'click' to indicate appropriate reconnection but requires more dexterity. A secondary disconnection point in the tubing further away from the point of insertion is sometimes available and is useful for difficult-to-access insertion sites.

Reservoirs

There are different reservoir sizes. The larger 3 ml size is useful for children with a higher insulin requirement, to avoid more frequent reservoir changes. The standard 1.5-2 ml size is applicable to most children, as it can hold sufficient insulin to last three days and allows the reservoir to be changed at the same time as the rest of the infusion set.

Connecting the pump with the insulin

1- Draw the insulin into the reservoir: This is similar to drawing up a vial with a syringe. Room temperature insulin makes drawing up without air bubbles easier.
2- Air bubbles must be expelled.
3- The tubing should be connected to the reservoir.
4- Prime the tubing: Pumps have a mechanism to prime the tubing with insulin and ensure the pump's piston head (that pushes insulin out of the reservoir) is firmly pressed against the reservoir plunger.

5- Again, air bubbles must be expelled.
6- Connect the pump and prime the cannula: Attach the pump tubing to the cannula. Pumps have an automated feature to fill the small amount of dead space in the cannula. Alternatively, a manual bolus may be needed to fill-in the dead space. The exact amount varies with cannula type (0.1–1 unit), check the manufacturer booklet.
7- Now that the pump is connected. Some pumps come with a belt clip or pouch with a clip that allows them to be worn on trousers. A wide range of accessories is available, including pouches and garters, to fit different pumps. Thigh pouches can be used to hold the pump. A small hole cut into a trouser pocket to feed the tubing through can be considered.
8- Some devices have remote-control options to control the pump if worn in a difficult-to-access place.
9- Patch pumps: Although there is no or only very short tubing in patch pumps, priming and inserting the pump is still applicable. The priming and insertion processes are often more automated. No disconnection is usually needed. When wearing a patch pump, it is important to consider that it will be in place for up to three days, so we should select a site that is suitable for the next few days' activities.

Sites for cannula insertion

As long as the new site is at least 2-2.5 cm away from the previous site, avoiding the waistband and 2.5 cm from the umbilicus, any orientation preferred by the patient can be used. Figure 2.1 shows some examples.

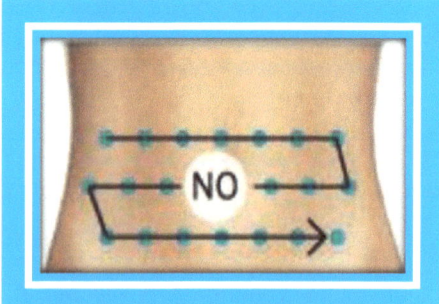

Figure 2.1

Helpful points to remember:

1- Anaesthetic creams can be used to reduce discomfort.
2- Adhesive sprays can be used to improve the security of the cannula.

3- For older children, shaving the desired site ensures proper contact with the cannula adhesive and reduces risk of slippage.
4- Barrier dressings can be used to prevent allergy.
5- Slight stinging after insertion can be normal, but if this persists beyond 30 minutes and especially with movement, removal and reinsertion of the cannula is suggested, as discomfort may indicate that the cannula is inserted in a muscle.
6- Bleeding into the cannula lumen suggests that the cannula may be positioned in or near a blood vessel and may need to be removed as insulin absorption may be different.
7- Problems with setting up and wearing the pump are one of the leading causes of unexplained high blood glucose on pumps.

Making the Transition

As excited as patients are to get the new pump, there may be a hint of fear when transitioning to a new form of therapy. To make transition to insulin pump as easy as possible for your patients, you need to offer support and encouragement and make sure you can work together with your patients and nurses during transition period.

Learning all they can about the pump prior to starting to use it can be helpful and ease some of their fears. They need to practice using the pump before putting it on. They can carry their pump around with them for a few days and practise giving boluses without being connected, or by being connected, but using saline instead of insulin.
Diabetes healthcare providers need to explain to the child and their family the process of setting up the pump and putting it on, and make sure to answer any questions or concerns.

Allow your patient to try it

Saline pump trials offer useful opportunities to evaluate suitability for pump treatment and may be a useful additional educational way to allow the pump user to address, and potentially alleviate, any concerns regarding wearing the pump. It also involves an intensive period of learning during which errors may occur.

An initial period of worsening glucose control can happen, and this may be a cause of frustration for a new pump user, therefore support in the initiation phase of pump treatment is extremely important to explore people's expectations prior to pump therapy. That's why your patient expectations must be realistic and achievable to avoid frustration and disengagement.

What to consider during pump initiation

For optimized pump initiation, the following should be considered:

A- Saline trials where indicated (additional educational way).

B- Initiation sessions: Can take 2–4 hours of intensive and focused training by a specialist diabetes educator. Training can be done in groups or one-to-one. Continuous support and follow-up are also needed.

If appropriate, more than one person from the family should be trained. Education should be provided on:
1- Setting up the pump: drawing up insulin, inserting cannulas, setting changes, and troubleshooting.
2- Infusion set insertion and changing.
3- Using the pump: basal, bolus, temporary basal, main functions, suspending pump and changing general settings.
4- Managing carbohydrate counting.
5- Using bolus advisor.
6- Managing hypo- and hyperglycaemia with pump and troubleshooting.

Written information should be provided on the above, including contact numbers for the on-call support team if possible.

C- Support: Patients and their family should be provided with contact details of diabetes specialist nurses, pump companies and other helpful contacts (e.g. online resources). A follow-up date and plan should be agreed to ensure correct usage, provide further education and to correct any problems. More close monitoring and support may be needed for children with reduced hypoglycaemia awareness and recurrent or severe hypoglycaemia.

D- Dose adjusting of long-acting insulin the day before starting pump therapy:
1- If taken in the evening, reduce your child's long-acting insulin dose by 50% the evening before.
2- If taken in the morning, omit the dose of long-acting insulin on the day when you are initiating pump therapy. Give the child fast-acting insulin with carbohydrates (CHO) for breakfast and correct any high blood glucose levels.

E- Frequent follow up and support is required initially as follows:
1- Daily telephone follow-up with diabetes/pump nurse for the initial 1–2 weeks.
2- Set change at day three.

3- Review on day seven to consider dose adjustment.
4- Within first 2 weeks, carry out basal rate testing for 24 h period and make appropriate adjustments.
5- Within 1 month, diabetes/pump nurse follow-up in clinic.
6- First review in pump clinic usually within 1-2 months after starting pump therapy, then a minimum of four times a year if stable.

During follow up there are additional points to focus on shown (see pump follow-up section).

2.2 Basal rate calculation and setting

The basal (background) rate is the rate at which the insulin pump gives doses of insulin continually over a 24-hour period. This basal rate is responsible for about 25-50% of the child's daily insulin requirement. But it is important that higher basal rates are NOT used to mask the failure to bolus with all CHO. It is necessary to get the basal rate right, therefore, children under five may require only 20-30% of the new total daily dose as a total basal rate. Theoretically, if the basal rate is correct the patient could fast all day and their blood glucose level would remain more or less stable (5-8 mmol/l).

Children with diabetes will need approximately 20-30% less insulin on a pump than their present requirements on pen injections; this will depend on three major factors (age, HbA1c levels and frequency of hypos).

Table 2.4: How to calculate the hourly basal rate

Steps	Example
1- What is the average total fast-acting insulin in 24 hours?	26 units
2- How much long-acting insulin do they need in 24 hours?	22 units
3- For total daily dose add together 1+2 to give the pre-pump total daily dose.	26 + 22 = 48 units
4- Subtract 25-30% from the pre-pump total daily dose to get the total daily pump dose.	70% of 48units = 33.6 units
5- Total 24 hr basal rate: Advise your patients what percentage of the pre-pump total dose should be subtracted.	33.6/2 = 16.8 units/24 hours
6- Hourly basal rate Three options can be used to divide the total 24-hour basal rate into an hourly one. Choose the most suitable option for your patient.	16.8/24 = 0.7 units/hour

a- Divide the total basal rate into 24 equal parts. b- Divide the basal rate into blocks of time giving more insulin per hour early morning and afternoon/evening. c- Use pump company calculator. This uses different profiles for different age ranges and mimics the body's natural variation in insulin levels over 24 hours.	

Ensure a correct and safe starting dose

Ensuring a smooth transition to pump therapy helps to build up the confidence of both healthcare professionals and patients, therefore it is important that the dose of the basal rate is not too high to reduce the risk of hypoglycaemia.

Different basal rates can be initiated for different situations.
1. The body often produces more insulin in the early morning and early evenings; however, a flat basal rate is usually programmed to start with, and then adjustments can be made at these times as indicated.
2. The older the child, the higher the basal rate required, in general, and between 2 and 6 Am particularly.
3. The pump has the ability to deliver different basal rates over 24 hours. Most children with diabetes have between four and six different basal rates. These will be determined according to individual needs over the first few weeks.
4. If there are obvious patterns of insulin resistance or sensitivity, such as waking with hyperglycaemia or hypoglycaemia at night, then divide 24 hours into 4 or 5 blocks for more effective treatment.

Different basal rates over 24 hours

Example 1: A 6-year-old boy who is on MDI with a TDDi of 26 units: 30% reduction = 18.2 units If a 50% basal rate is required, then divide by 2 = 9.1 units basal rate over 24 hours			
Time	Units/hour	Total (units)	24-hour total (units)
00:00–03:00	0.37	1.11	

03:00–08:00	0.4	2.0	
08:00–15:00	0.35	2.45	
15:00–19:00	0.3	1.2	
19:00–00:00	0.37	1.85	8.61

Example 2: A 3-year-old girl who is on MDI with a TDDi of 11 units:
25% reduction = 8.25 units
If a 50% basal rate is required, then divide by 2 = 4.12 units basal rate over 24 hours.

Time	Units/hour	Total (units)	24-hour total (units)
00:00–07:00	0.175	1.225	
07:00–12:00	0.175	0.875	
12:00–18:00	0.15	0.9	
18:00–00:00	0.15	0.9	3.9

Example 3: A 13-year-old boy who is on MDI with a TDDi of 64 units:
25% reduction = 48 units
If a 50% basal rate is required, then divide by 2 = 24 units basal rate over 24 hours. There is more than one answer.
Answer 1

Time	Units/hour	Total (units)	24-hour total (units)
00:00–04:00	1.0	4.0	
04:00–08:00	1.2	4.8	
08:00–12:00	1.0	4.0	

12:00–16:00	1.0	4.0	
16:00–20:00	0.8	3.2	
20:00-00:00	1.0	4.0	24

Example 3: A 13-year-old boy who is on MDI with a TDDi of 64 units:
25% reduction = 48 units
If a 50% basal rate is required, then divide by 2 = 24 units basal rate over 24 hours.
Answer 2

Time	Units/hour	Total (units)	24-hour total (units)
00:00–04:00	1.0	4.0	
04:00–08:00	1.0	4.0	
08:00–12:00	1.0	4.0	
12:00–16:00	1.0	4.0	
16:00–20:00	1.0	4.0	
20:00-00:00	1.0	4.0	24

Example 3: A 13-year-old boy who is on MDI with a TDDi of 64 units:
25% reduction = 48 units
If a 50% basal rate is required, then divide by 2 = 24 units basal rate over 24 hours.
Answer 3

Time	Calculation	Total (units)	24-hour total (units)
00:00–04:00	1.0	4.0	
04:00–07:00	1.0	3.0	
07:00–10:00	1.0	3.0	

10:00–18:00	1.0	8.0	
18:00–00:00	1.0	6.0	24

Refining the calculated basal rate

The child with diabetes in Example 3, Answer 3, has a calculated basal rate of 1.0 units/h. If he is at risk of overnight hypoglycaemia and dawn phenomenon, the calculated basal rate can be modified by making a 10-20% reduction or increment, as shown in Table 2.5.

Table 2.5 The calculated basal rate

Time	Calculation	Basal settings (per hour)
00:00–04:00	1.0 − (1.0 × 0.2) = 0.8	0.8 units
04:00–07:00	1.0 + (1.0 × 0.2) = 1.2	1.2 units
07:00–10:00	1.0	1.0 units
10:00–18:00	1.0 − (1.0 × 0.1) = 0.9	0.9 units
18:00–00:00	1.0 + (1.0 × 0.2) = 1.2	1.2 units

These durations indicate that there is significant inter- and intra-individual variation that may alter the action of insulin. Adjustments in basal rates to take into account usual circadian rhythm, activity and meal patterns.

Calculated insulin requirements from injection dosages may be higher if there is low risk of hypoglycaemia and if the starting HbA_{1c} is high. With experience, the reduction in TDDi can be lowered to account for this. However, a higher reduction in TDDi may be needed if there is a high risk of hypoglycaemia, loss of hypoglycaemia awareness or a history of severe disabling hypoglycaemia. Some basal feature of the pump are shown on table9

Some software packages will calculate initial circadian basal infusion rates. These are based on physiological data and fine tuning is likely to be needed.

Table 2.6 Quick-acting insulin pharmacokinetics

	Onset	Duration	Peak
Analogue insulin (e.g. aspart, lispro and glulisine)	15 min	2–5 h	50–90 min

| Soluble human insulin | 30 min | Up to 8 h | 2–4 h |

2.3 Insulin to carbohydrate ratio calculation

Insulin to carbohydrate ratio (ICR) is a ratio that specifies the number of grams of carbohydrate covered by each unit of rapid- or short-acting insulin. An ICR tells us how many units of insulin your patient needs to cover a specified number of CHO grams (g). For example, if their ratio is 1:15, your patient will need one unit of insulin for every 15 g of CHO he/she eats. They may already have calculated an ICR when on MDI. This can be used in your pump settings and you may need to consider different ICR at different times of the day. ICR allows more accurate bolus dose calculations and it should be regularly reviewed as the child grows and develops.

Calculating ICR

Calculate your patient's total daily dose and subtract 20-30% (as demonstrated in Table 2.4), then divide 300 by the figure (for preschool children), or divide 500 by this figure (for ages 5 years and above). This will vary every day, so use an average value from a typical day. Add together both their total background amount and food/correction boluses. If already on a pump don't reduce by 20-30%.

How to calculate ICR:
A- If your patient is not on the pump:
    500 divided by total daily dose
    (300 divided by daily total dose for preschool children)
B- If your patient is on insulin pump:
Step 1: 75% of daily total dose. (Divide the daily total dose by 100 then multiply by 75.)
Step 2: ICR = 500 divided by 75% of total daily dose.

Example 1: An 11-year-old child who is on MDI with a TDDi of 20 units.

(20 units/100) x 75 = 15 units

500/15 units = 33.3 g

This means they will need approximately 1 unit of insulin for every 33.3 g of CHO.

Example 2- A 3-year-old girl who is on MDI with a TDDi of 11 units:	Example 3- A 13-year-old boy who is on MDI with a TDDi of 64 units:
25% reduction = 8.25 units	25% reduction = 48 units
'300 rule' (preschool children)	'500 rule' (children aged 5 and over)
'300 rule': 300/8.25 = 36.3 ICR is 1:36.3 or 36 g. This means that 1 unit of insulin is required for every 36 g of carbohydrate consumed	'500 rule': 500/24 = 20.83 Round to 20 g carbohydrate ICR is 1:20 This means that 1 unit of insulin is required for every 20 g of carbohydrate consumed

As it is known that patients require less insulin while using a pump, they also need less insulin for food they eat, therefore their ICR is higher.

ICR can be influenced by the following factors:
1- Time of day: the need for insulin is often highest in the morning (at breakfast) and the ratio may need to be higher, e.g. 1:8 instead of 1:10.
2- Physical activity: children may need less insulin during and after activities. For example, you may need to change their ratio from 1:10 to 1:15 during and after activity.
3- Illness and infection: more insulin is often needed during illness and infections, so you may need to increase the basal rate and look at increasing the ratio. Episodes of severe vomiting and diarrhoea may require less insulin. Temporary basal rate may need to be considered in such situations.
4- Periods of rapid growth and puberty require higher insulin and lower ICR.
5- Menstrual periods: girls often need more insulin the day before or during their period.

The healthcare team should be able to offer advice specific to individual circumstances. Some basal features of the pump are shown in Table 2.7.

Table 2.7 Basal features on pumps

Basal profiles	You can use different profiles for days with different levels of activity or insulin requirements. For example, profiles may be set for weekends and weekdays, to manage premenstrual hormonal changes and during illness.

Temporary basal rate	Can be used to increase or decrease the basal rate for short periods (0–24 h). This is useful to adapt dynamically to circumstances, for example, during exercise, stress or illness.

How much bolus you need to give with meals

Most insulin pumps have insulin bolus calculators integrated into them, which will calculate an insulin dose to match ingested food and to correct hyperglycaemia. Bolus insulin dose is calculated based on individual ICR, insulin sensitivity factor and glucose target.

The ICR is programmed into the pump. Many people need more insulin for a given amount of carbohydrate at breakfast. Therefore, you may need to programme different ICRs for different times.

2.4 Correction dose calculation

A correction dose is an extra amount of fast-acting insulin that is recommended in order to keep blood glucose levels within a target range (usually 5-8 mmol/l / 90-140 mg/dl). Sometimes referred to as an Insulin Sensitivity Factor (ISF) and is. You can work this out from the total amount of insulin injected each day. The correction dose required depends on your patient's insulin sensitivity.

Correction Bolus Formula:

(Current BG - Target BG) ÷ ISF = units of insulin

This can be estimated using the '100 rule' if using mmol/L or the '1800 rule' if using mg/dl for glucose measurements, as shown in Table 2.8. This will predict how much one unit of fast-acting insulin will lower the child's blood glucose when it's high.

Table 2.8 How to calculate ISF

'100 rule': for mmol/l	'1800 rule': for mg/dl
If you are using mmol/l meter: 100 divided by total daily insulin dose (TDDi) on insulin pump	If you using mg/dl meter: 1800 divided by TDDi on insulin pump
Example: TDDi 50 units 100/50= 2 mmol/l ISF is 1:2. i.e. you need 1 unit of insulin to bring blood glucose down by 2	Example: TDDi 50 units 1800/50 = 36 mg/dl ISF is 1:36 mg/dl. i.e. you need 1 unit of insulin to bring the blood glucose down

| mmol/l. | by 36 mg/dl. |

When correcting high blood glucose levels at mealtimes, you should aim to bring your patient's blood glucose down to 7 mmol/l or 126 mg/dl; this will take about two to three hours.

The correction dose will need to be tested regularly. As the child grows and develops the amount of insulin required to correct high blood glucose should be increased.

To avoid insulin stacking, which can cause a hypo, avoid insulin correction more frequently than once every 2 hours. Most pumps have a built-in mechanism which prevents stacking by calculating active insulin in your patient's body.

Your patient's correction dose may also vary through the night, often needing less insulin to lower blood glucose. Always be cautious when correcting at night. ISF may also need fine-tuning if hypo- or hyperglycaemia is recurrent after meals or after glucose corrections.

Blood glucose targets

It's important for blood glucose levels to stay in a healthy range. Blood glucose targets vary from individual to individual. Different targets can be set for different times to ensure optimal personalised glucose control. The target you set will be used by the pump to work out the amount of insulin needed when using its bolus advisor.

Insulin on-board (IOB) and active insulin time

IOB is the calculation that tells you how much insulin is still active in your body from previous bolus doses. Most typically, it is set at 4 hours and it is set to ensure the bolus calculator can estimate the 'on board' or 'active' insulin. It can be increased or decreased to address recurrent hypo- or hyperglycaemia after correction or after meals doses.
Everyone is different, and their bodies may absorb insulin at different rates. Furthermore, children's insulin absorption may vary from week-to-week or day-to-day.

Shorter IOB times mean the pump will only include the effect of more recent insulin administered and there is a risk of underestimating insulin on board. This can result in insulin 'stacking', where a bolus acts in addition to a previous bolus, which will result in lower-than-desired glucose levels and a higher risk of hypoglycaemia. This is why it is appropriate to set this feature for 4 hours, or longer for someone with increased risk of hypoglycaemia.

If the IOB is set for a duration of over 4 hours, then the effect of insulin on board may be overestimated, resulting in smaller boluses and higher-than-desired glucose concentrations.

The active insulin time should be increased in small children and children with impaired kidney function, as up to 75% of insulin is cleared by the kidneys. It also changes with the insulin type and dose.

Different bolus options

Boluses can be delivered in three ways: standard or normal bolus; square-wave or extended bolus; and multi-wave or dual-wave bolus, as shown in Table 2.9.

Table 2.9 Different bolus types

Standard or normal bolus (Bolus insulin is delivered immediately)	Used for correction (similar to bolus insulin injection) or normal meal.
Extended or square-wave bolus (Bolus insulin is delivered over an extended, defined period of time).	Used for high fat meals, which slow the absorption of carbohydrate (such as pizza or curry) and low glycaemic index foods, such as porridge.
Multi-wave or dual-wave bolus (A combination of extended bolus and normal bolus).	Used for large carbohydrate meals or separate courses and for delays in digestion such as from gastroparesis.

Using dual- or multi-wave boluses:
1. Make sure the Dual/ Square Wave option is on.
2. Select On, then press ACT
3. Calculate your food and/or correction bolus amount
4. Select Dual Wave Bolus, then press ACT
5. Enter the desired amount for the total dual bolus units

Use the pump bolus calculator or manually calculate the total bolus required.
Determine the time period for the extended bolus (this is usually 2–4 h but may be longer). Divide the bolus into the percentage to be given immediately. The remainder will be given over a longer period of time.

It is important to remember that the temporary basal feature cannot be used while dual- or multi-wave bolus is operating and the bolus can be stopped at any time

2.5 Pump technical issues/failure

Parents need to keep a written record of their child's pump basal rate and bolus ratio for each hour in case the pump fails and they need to go back to injections.

What should we do when our patient's pump isn't working properly and they need to go back to MDI?
1- Parents/patients should contact the pump manufacturer, who may arrange to supply another pump.
2- Use their usual correction doses and ICR. Deliver the fast-acting insulin (pen or syringe). Patients will probably need more corrections than usual.
3- If the pump manufacturer can't get a replacement pump within 24 hours, calculate your patients' total daily basal rate on the pump and inject this amount immediately as long-acting insulin (glargine, detemir or degludec).
E.g. If they are on a 24-hour basal rate of 25 units, inject 25 units of long-acting insulin. Close monitoring is advised as this dose may need to be increased. This should be continued until they receive the replacement pump.
4- On recommencing the pump, the long-acting insulin will still have some effect for 24-40 hours, so a 10-25% temporary basal rate reduction is needed.

2.6 Removing the pump

Sometimes children need to remove their pump, for example, when they go swimming, have showers or take part in contact sports (such as rugby or boxing). Although new pumps are waterproof, many children feel uncomfortable keeping the pump attached while swimming.

When removing the pump, the following precautions need to be taken:
1- If the pump is removed for up to two hours, blood glucose needs to be checked before and during removal, and when pump is reconnected.
2- If the pump is removed for more than two hours, blood glucose should be checked and food and correction boluses given by injection, or pump should be reconnected to give appropriate insulin every two hours using normal bolus.
3- If the pump is removed for more than 24 hours, long-acting insulin will be needed.

Notes: Removing the pump for more than two hours may cause hyperglycaemia later, due to missed basal insulin, so patients should continue to monitor blood glucose for several hours following reconnection of the pump. In the case of exercise, less insulin may be needed (see exercise and activity chapter). Advise your patients to keep the pump in a safe place.

2.7 Temporary basal rates

The insulin pump also enables a temporary basal insulin rate to be set, and this is most commonly used for exercise or during illness. You can set more than one temporary basal program.
This feature is not automatic. You have to choose how much less or more basal insulin you want (usually as a percentage of your normal basal rate) and for how long. The insulin pump will later automaticly return to the original basal rate pattern after the set period of time.

2.8 Keeping your emergency kit ready

Emergency kit should be carried at all times for emergency use dnd it should contain:
      1- Fast-acting insulin pen or syringe and insulin
      2- Hypo treatment (hypo remedies, Glucogel or Glucotablet)
      3- Blood glucose and ketone testing kit
      4- Spare cannula
      5- Spare insulin vial
      6- Spare batteries
      7- Spare infusion line and reservoir

2.9 Pump follow-up and support

Initially, patients and their families require close support by diabetes healthcare providers. Ongoing advice and support is needed. This can be achieved through clinic visits, telephone, video or e-mail contact. The frequency of follow-up sessions may vary depending on clinical need, but initially they should be every 1-2 weeks, then at least four times a year.

The first day after starting to use the pump, patients need check glucose 2-hourly and continue this overnight.

They need to correct blood glucose so that it is maintained at <14 mmol/L or <250 mg/dl with a correction bolus as advised. They also need to treat blood glucose <4 mmol/L or <70 mg/dl.

Recording or downloading blood glucose readings is important and helps the team to make correct decisions and make appropriate dose changes. A suggested example of clinic follow-up and monitoring protocol is shown in Table 2.10.

Table 2.10 follow up and monitoring protocol

First day after pump start	1-Check glucose two-hourly and continue this overnight. 2- Treat blood glucose <4 mmol/L or <70 mg/dl. 3- Correct blood glucose >14 mmol/L or >250 mg/dl with a correction bolus as advised. Check ketones. 4- Record blood glucose readings.
Initial 1-2 weeks	1- Continue as above. 2- Record blood glucose readings or download pump/glucose meter readings. 3- Daily telephone follow-up with diabetes/pump nurse. 4- Carry out basal rate testing for 24 h period and make appropriate adjustments.
Day 3	Set change.
Day 7	Review on day 7 to consider dose adjustment.
One month	Follow-up in pump clinic: 8- Review Hypoglycaemia and DKA prevention guidelines. 9- Check 3am glucose at least once during the month. 10- Check 2-hour post-meal blood glucose for all meals on a given day.
Two months	Second review in pump clinic usually 2 months after starting pump therapy, then a minimum of four times a year if stable.
Every three months	1- Patient needs to visit their healthcare provider, even if they feel well and their blood glucose values are within target range. 2- Review blood glucose downloads and insulin pump settings with your patient. 3- Make sure HbA1c test done. 4- Provide further education 5- Review the clinical, glucose meter and pump data. 6- Set further goals. 7- Ensure pump is working appropriately. 8- Inspect cannula sites. 9- Consider ordering supplies and consumables. 10- Discuss emergencies and possible technical difficulties. 11- Provide information on how to download pump data.
Annually for children ≥ 10 years and	1- Dilated eye exam by a qualified ophthalmologist. 2- Foot examination (inspection, touch, pain, position and vibration sensation). 3- Annual flu vaccination. 4- Regular dental visits.

twice yearly for children younger than 10 years	5- Diabetes education review (including exercise, driving, puberty and drugs). 6- Replace glucagon kit (with new prescription from physician). 7- Transition review. **LABORATORY TESTS:** 1- Test HbA1c four or more times a year. 2- HDL, LDL, triglyceride, TFT, celiac screen yearly. 3- Microalbuminuria and albumin/creatinine ratio yearly.
Every visit:	1- Weight, height and BP check. 2- Review goals for blood glucose, meal plan and exercise.
Every day:	1- Check blood glucose 4-6 times a day and always before bed. 2- Test before exercise and have a fast-acting carbohydrate with you when you exercising. 3- If your blood glucose is above 14 mg/dl twice in a row, take an injection and change the infusion set.

Encourage your patients and their families to:
1. Check the infusion site and tubing at least daily.
2. Change the site every 2–3 days to reduce risk of infection and degradation of insulin in hot temperatures.
3. Clean the insertion site to allow good adhesion and shave if necessary.
4. Rotate their cannula site regularly.
5. If in doubt, redraw new insulin into a new reservoir and perform a set change (attach new tubing and insert a new cannula).
6. Always have access to a spare reservoir, infusion sets, insulin and batteries at all times (even for day trips).
7. Record and review their bolus, basal, carbohydrate, blood sugar and activity in log sheets. Alternatively, these data can be automatically logged in pumps, or even Smartphone apps, and downloaded.

3 Managing clinical issues of pump therapy

3.1 Managing pump therapy
3.2 Hypoglycaemia
3.3 Hyperglycaemia
3.4 Presence of ketones
3.5 Diabetic ketoacidosis and illness
3.6 Testing and adjusting basal rate
3.7 Testing and adjusting insulin to carbohydrate ratio
3.8 Continuous glucose monitoring
3.9 Meter/pump downloads, interpretation of blood glucose readings and decision making
3.10 Using CGM to manage difficult diabetes cases
3.11 Coming off the pump

3.1 Managing pump therapy

General rules for adjusting insulin dose:

1- If the change occurs before a meal or at night (during sleep) it can be attributed to the basal rate.
2- If the change occurs within two to four hours after a meal, it is most likely due to the bolus before that meal.
3- Make small adjustments initially to evaluate your patient's response to the change, especially when increasing doses at night time. This is to ensure that your decision is correct and to keep your patient from experiencing hypoglycaemia.
4- In the beginning, it is advised to set the target blood glucose a little higher than ideal and accept greater fluctuation in blood glucose values than usual until the patient adjusts to wearing the pump and is comfortable with its use.
5- The goal is not to raise blood glucose more than 2.8 mmol/L (or 50 mg/dl) two hours after a meal. The meal bolus is based on the insulin to carbohydrate ratio (one unit of insulin to a determined number of grams of carbohydrate).
6- Raise or lower the number of grams of carbohydrate covered by one unit of insulin. Make small adjustments: 1 to 2 grams of carbohydrate for each adjustment.
   For example, if the insulin to carbohydrate ratio is 1:15 and the blood glucose two hours after is well above the pre-meal blood glucose, adjust ICR to 1:13.
7- The next step is fine-tuning the insulin pump parameters. It is a three-part process and may take up to a week for each part. The three parts are: testing and adjusting the basal rate, testing and adjusting the meal bolus and testing and adjusting the correction bolus. The three weeks shouldn't be consecutive and can be scheduled for the convenience of you and the patient.
8- Ensure choosing times when you will be available to phone the patient/parents to work with them on insulin adjustments. You may also schedule clinic visits to fine-tune the insulin pump parameters.

3.2 Hypoglycaemia

Definition: hypoglycaemia is commonly called a "hypo" and means low blood glucose. It is defined as a blood glucose level less than 4 mmol/l (or 72 mg/dl) and should be treated. Maintaining your patient's blood glucose no lower than this allows time for them to recognize any symptoms and take the necessary action.

The most common causes of hypos are:

a- Giving too much insulin (i.e. more insulin than required) which can be due to overestimation of carbohydrate (CHO) content of food, by mistake or if the child decides not to finish his calculated meal.

b- Physical activity: unplanned or underestimated activity in terms of time and intensity.
c- Alcohol: excessive alcohol can cause hypoglycaemia.

When assessing your patients for the causes of hypoglycaemia you need to ask two main questions:
1- What blood glucose level do they count as a hypo?
2- At what level do they notice warning symptoms when they experience a hypo?
3- Gold score or Clarke score

What are the clues to night-time hypoglycaemia?
Even if your patient can not measure their blood glucose at night there are clues that indicate if they go low at night:
1- They wake up feeling confused and complain of headaches.
2- Their morning blood glucose fluctuates from high to low.

However, these symptoms may be absent, and the only way to know if hypos are happening is by testing. Consider night-time glucose testing or a continuous glucose monitor (see CGM section).

A hypoglycaemic episode during the previous 12- 24 hours may increase the risk of further episodes and can also lead to unpredictable blood glucose levels over the next 12- 24 hours due to the body releasing various hormones in response to hypoglycaemia.

Common symptoms of hypoglycaemia

Young children may not be able to tell you how they feel during hypoglycaemia, even during times of rapid glucose change. Therefore, carers need to observe for any symptoms or signs children with diabetes may experience. These symptoms are very important and should never be ignored, even if the CGM monitor suggests a stable or normal glucose. Diabetes technology can be inaccurate and may be incorrect, so it is important to validate symptoms using a capillary glucose measurement.

Parents need to recognise their child's signs of hypos, and the terms they use to describe them.

The commonest signs are:
a. going pale
b. shakiness
c. being unusually quiet

d. sweating
   e. becoming confused or aggressive
   f. loss of consciousness
   g. fits (rare)

Remember that the younger the child, the vaguer the symptoms, and hypos can be difficult to recognise in children younger than two years old.

Insulin pump and hypoglycaemia

The risk of hypoglycaemia is still present, even when using an insulin pump (for the same reasons as MDI). However, because pump therapy only uses fast-acting insulin and you can control the delivery, we have more ways of dealing with and preventing a hypoglycaemia.

Hypoglycaemia prevention and management

I- **Prevention**

To prevent and treat hypoglycaemia, it's essential to understand the effect of insulin doses and types; food types and CHO content; exercise duration and intensity. The combination of the latter three elements will determine your patient's glucose level.

1- Check the insulin to carbohydrate ratio (ICR) and ensure it is correct – it may differ at different times of the day. Consider testing ICR.
2- Calculate CHO correctly to ensure correct bolus.
3- Consider splitting bolus or using different type/duration of bolus if larger amounts of CHO or slowly absorbed meals are eaten.
4- When giving correction boluses, work out how much is needed. Although most pumps include insulin on board in bolus calculation, fast-acting insulin may last in the body for up to five hours so it's advisable to correct no more frequently than two-hourly.
5- Always look for a pattern before changing basal, food bolus or correction bolus. Wherever possible, use insulin pump decision-making tools (Bolus Wizard, EZ Carb, and Bolus Advisor etc.).
6- Ideally, basal rates should be tested every one to two months, but at least every three months to make sure they are correct.
7- Use a temporary reduction of basal rate when exercising.
8- Avoid insulin stacking, encourage giving bolus through the wizard.

II- **Management**

The first step is to check whether it is the basal rate or the bolus which is incorrect and needs adjustment.

The following two factors suggest that it is the type or amount of bolus rate that needs adjustment:
1- A large bolus given as a one-off standard bolus rather than as dual wave.
2- Hypo within four hours of the last bolus.

Consider the type of food: does it contain slow-release CHO?

The following two factors suggest that it is the basal rate needs adjustment:
1- Hypos at night or at least 3-5 hours after the last bolus. (A bolus of fast-acting insulin usually only lasts 4 hours).
2- Repeated episodes of hypo at similar times of the day/night.

The following factors suggest that both basal and bolus need to be considered:
1- Exercise, particularly if lasting more than 30-60 minutes, can produce hypos 24-36 hours after finishing.
2- Wrong calculation of basal and correction ratio.

You may need to reduce the bolus both before and after exercise and reduce the basal rate for up to 36 hours.
If you are unsure, ask parents to keep detailed records of glucose levels and discuss with your patient/parents.

Table 3.1 shows severity, symptoms and treatment of hypoglycaemia.

Table 3.1 hypoglycaemia severity, symptoms and treatment

Hypo severity	Symptoms	Treatment
Mild	• Pale • Sweating • Shaky/wobbly • Hungry • Tired or sleepy • Headache • Lack of concentration	Give 5-15gm sugar carbohydrate depending on the child's age and sensitivity e.g.: 1. 2-4 Glucose tablets=150ml Coke OR 1-3 jelly babies OR ½-1 ½ tubes Glucogel. 2. Recheck blood glucose in 15 minutes and retreat if BG<4 mmol/L. 3. If more than 30 minutes to next meal, give 15-20 gm starchy CHO snack to hold blood glucose, e.g. slice of toast or 2 digestive biscuits.

Moderate	• Irritable • Dizzy • Headache • Blurred vision • Too confused to eat or drink • Unsteady on feet • Slurred speech	1. If able to eat/drink treat as for mild hypo (above). 2. If uncooperative but able to swallow give Glucogel. 3. Recheck blood glucose in 15 minutes and retreat if BG <4 mmol/L. 4. If more than 30 minutes to next meal, give 15-20 gm starchy CHO snack e.g. slice of toast or 2 digestive biscuits.
Severe	• Semi-conscious or unconscious • Convulsion/seizure	1. Turn child onto side and do not give anything by mouth as this may cause choking. 2. Give Glucagon injection 0.5mg if <12 years or <25kg. 1mg if >12 years old or >25kg. 3. If you cannot give the injection call for an ambulance. 4. When child is conscious follow steps 1-3 for mild hypo. 5. Monitor blood glucose readings every 15 minutes for at least an hour as it is not uncommon for blood glucose readings to fall again.

Be aware that:

1- When treating hypoglycaemia with fruit juice, you may need double the CHO to get the same effect as other treatments due to the slower absorption rate of fructose.

2- Long-acting CHO is no longer routinely recommended in addition to a hypo treatment, as it can lead to over-treatment and highs later. However, a maximum of 20 g may be considered in certain circumstances, like pre- and post-exercise, insulin overdose and if your patient has had a hypo during the last 24 hours, or if you are at all unsure.

3. For an effective treatment for hypos, chocolate is NOT recommended because the presence of fat further slows the rate of absorption and it takes longer to break down the lactose found in milk than it does glucose.

4. If your patient becomes unconscious due to severe hypoglycaemia, a glucagon injection should be given to raise the glucose level and an ambulance should be called. Ask your patients/parents to regularly check that their child's glucagon is in date and that they always take it on holiday with them.

What is negative correction?

A patient might need to calculate a BG bolus even if the BG is lower than target and they are planning to eat. In this case, the BG bolus might be a negative number. This number will tell you how much to reduce the carbohydrate bolus. Basically, taking less insulin than they would normally take for the food they are planning to eat. This is often referred to as a negative correction (see example below).

> **Example:**
> If patient's ISF is 1: 3 mmol/l and their target BG is 6.0 mmol/l how much is their BG bolus if your BG is 4.5 mmol/l?
>
> 4.5 mmol/L (BG) – 6.0 mmol/L (target BG) = -1.5 (mmol/L lower than target)
> -1.5 (mmol/L lower than target) ÷ 3.0 mmol/L (ISF) =- 0.50 units.
>
> In this example, you would subtract 0.50 units from the carbohydrate bolus to get the bolus total.
>
> If your carbohydrate bolus was 5.50 units, you would only bolus 5.00 units (5.50 minus 0.50).
>
> It is important to treat any blood sugar less than 4.0 mmol/L (or 72 mg/dl) with fast acting carbohydrates. In other words, eat or drink 15-20 grams of carbohydrate right away! In this case, after treating the low BG, you would then just take your usual carbohydrate bolus for the meal. Do not add the carbohydrates you used to treat the low BG into your calculation.

Common causes of hypoglycaemia and suggested solutions are shown in Table 3.2.

Table 3.2

Cause of hypoglycaemia	Solution
1- Too high basal rate.	Review and test basal rate regularly.
2- Too large bolus with food or different bolus type needed.	Use reduced or potentially multi-wave or extended bolus.
3- Over correction/frequent corrections (insulin stacking).	Avoid repeat bolus or use calculator.
4- Overestimating carbohydrates.	A- Review/refresh carbohydrate counting. B- Check insulin to carbohydrate ratios.
5- Infrequent blood glucose monitoring.	Test at least 4–6 times per day.
6- Inappropriate (too low) targets for blood glucose.	Adjust targets on bolus calculator.
7- Slow digestion.	Use multi-wave or extended bolus.

Treating hypoglycaemia

Training to enable prevention and self-management of hypoglycaemia should be provided to everyone with type 1 diabetes and to their families.

Children with diabetes and their carers should be advised as follows:
1- Consider suspending the pump and test before treating.
2- Take 15 grams of fast-acting carbohydrate and re-check blood glucose in 10–15 min.
3- If not corrected, repeat fast-acting carbohydrate and consider temporary basal reduction 10–20% (especially if recurrent or severe hypoglycaemia).
4- If unable to drink or unconscious, give glucagon injection and call ambulance.

3.3 Hyperglycaemia

Definition: Hyperglycaemia means high blood glucose. It occurs when the body does not have enough insulin or cannot use the insulin it has to turn glucose into energy. This is generally a glucose level higher than 14mmol/l (250 mg/dl), but some children may continue to be asymptomatic until even at higher values, such as 15-20 mmol/l (270-360 mg/dl).

Hyperglycaemia symptoms can include:
1. Thirst and passing a large amount of urine, day and night
2. Tiredness
3. Loss of weight
4. Feeling miserable and irritable, similar to hypo
5. Nausea and vomiting
6. Smelling of ketones (pear drops).

Test blood glucose to confirm, if vomiting, seek help immediately.

Causes of hyperglycaemia

A. Increased insulin requirements:
1. Reduced activity and exercise
2. Hormones (e.g. adrenaline and growth hormone)
3. Growth and increased body weight
4. Infection/illness: When you are unwell, your body is put under extra stress and often needs extra insulin to keep your blood glucose in the target range (see Sick Day Rules if you are unwell).
5. Stress

6. Steroids
7. Hot days: during summertime, insulin may be affected by the temperature, particularly if it is very hot. Not only is the air temperature high, but the insulin is close to your body constantly. If you are very warm, the insulin in the cartridge may be affected by the temperature and so not last as long as usual. This could lead to high blood glucose levels. It is advisable to change the cartridge more frequently during hot weather.

B. Insufficient insulin delivery:
1. Excessive CHO after hypo
2. Rebound following hypo
3. Forgot to give bolus or basal rate is too low
4. Pump stopped or forgot to reconnect pump
5. Bolus too little for the amount of CHO/under-calculated CHO content of food.

C. Pump causes
1. Empty cartridge
2. Pump failure and technical issues: although the pump performs many checks a day to ensure it is working, you need to make sure there is enough insulin in the pump, the battery is working and the pump is in RUN.
3. Alarms: The pump will alarm if there is a problem, such as an occlusion, and to warn you that the battery is running low or the insulin cartridge is running low. If these alarms are ignored (perhaps they happen during the night and are not heard), the pump runs out of insulin or the battery fails, you will not get the insulin you need, which will cause high blood glucose levels. The warning alarms for low battery or low cartridge insulin give you plenty of time to change sets and replace batteries if they are responded to promptly.

D. Infusion set causes
1. Left in too long: cannulas should be changed every 2 or 3 days depending on the type you are using. Sometimes they do not last quite as long as they should, which causes poor or variable absorption of the insulin so they need changing earlier. High blood glucose levels are a sign that the cannula may need changing sooner than is routine.
2. Insertion into a hardened area.
3. Inflammation at site.
4. Dislodged or blocked: remember that the insulin in the pump is rapid-acting insulin so, if there is a blockage or disconnection of the tubing or if the cannula has fallen out, the blood glucose will rise quickly.

5. Blood or large air bubble in tubing: it is important to make sure there are no air bubbles in your insulin cartridge when you change it and then check it every day to make sure no air bubbles have appeared. If they do, they can be primed out. If they are not spotted, there will be times when no insulin is being delivered, which will lead to high blood glucose levels.
6. Insulin leak.
7. Bent connector needles: take care when connecting and disconnecting your tubing to the cannula. If the needle inside the connector bends, this can prevent insulin being delivered properly.

Treatment of hyperglycaemia with insulin pumps

It can take up to 4 hours to normalize the blood sugar; however, if there is no improvement or worsening ketosis and high glucose, emergency medical assistance must be sought immediately. Causes of hyperglycaemia and treatment guidance are shown in Table 3.3.

Table 3.3

Issues	Suggested solutions
1. Cannula dislodgement	a- Ensure skin is adequately cleaned and prepared (including shaving if needed). b- Additional adhesive may be needed (sprays or dressing), especially if excessive sweating is the cause. c- If this is a recurrent problem, consider different cannula length or type. d- Ensure tugs on tubing are not a cause of this, in which case different length tubing could be helpful.
2. Tube breakage	Ensure tubing is not too long.
3. Air bubbles	a- Inspect tubing and reservoir. b- Keep insulin and infusion set at room temperature when filling and priming. c- Expel air bubbles if needed.
4. Site infection	a- Replace infusion set. b- Watch out for tenderness, redness, warmth, inflammation or swelling at the site of insertion. c- If fever, discharge, drainage, lump (abscess) are persisting features, seek medical attention.

5. Skin reaction to adhesive	Some children with sensitive skin may get redness, rash, itching and irritation with the cannula adhesive. This can be resolved by using a different adhesive type (if available), or a dressing under the adhesive (to prevent skin contact) with a larger, more suitable dressing over the site to secure the cannula.
6. Lumps at insertion site	a- Avoid lumpy sites. b- Rotate sites regularly. c- Lumps can also be caused by reaction to insulin, site infection (if other features, as above), incorrectly sited cannula or due to large insulin doses. Consider longer or shorter cannula.
7. High glucose before set change	a- May indicate prolonged set or reservoir use, change set earlier. b- Ensure infusion set and new insulin is drawn up more regularly, especially in hot environments.
8. Bolus or suspension due to accidental button presses	Rare, as most pumps feature alarms for insulin suspension and have safety features to prevent this (button lock-out and multiple steps needed).
9. Tube or cannula blockages	Most pumps will alarm if they can't deliver insulin (failed delivery alarm). Reservoir with fresh insulin and a set change usually corrects this. Rare but can happen with insulin crystals forming.
10. Pumps running out of insulin or batteries running down	Still considered as a common issue. Fill the reservoir with extra insulin.
11. Infection, illness, stress	See Sick Day Rules.
12. Basal rate too low or reduced activity	Increase basal insulin.
13. Insulin omission or insufficient insulin	Bolus to be taken 10- 15 min before meals; adjust ICR if needed.
14. Over treatment of hypoglycaemia	Review/refresh hypoglycaemia treatment.
15. Taking steroids	See Steroid section.
16. Pump failure	Contact pump company. Revert to injections and await

	replacement pump.

3.4 Presence of ketones

Our body's cells cannot use glucose for energy if there isn't sufficient insulin in our body. In this case, the cells will switch to an alternative source of energy and body fat will be broken down to produce energy.

The breakdown of fat can cause the build up of ketones. Eventually, the blood glucose and ketones rise to levels that cause acidosis, leading to diabetic ketoacidosis (DKA), which can be dangerous and will require hospital admission, particularly when associated with vomiting and dehydration. The only treatment for severe DKA is IV insulin and fluids because subcutaneous insulin does not work with poor circulation and cold, clammy skin.

Remember, now your patient is on a pump and they have no long-acting insulin, ketones can build up within four to five hours if there is insufficient insulin delivered. They will become unwell more quickly on a pump and action needs to be taken immediately. Checking blood glucose levels more frequently and at least six to eight times a day is therefore advisable to ensure early detection and management.

Blood ketones should be measured using a blood ketone meter. Patients should check the expiry date on blood strips before use. Testing for blood ketones is recommended If glucose levels are above 14 mmol/l (or 250 mg/dl).

Advise your patients to dispel ketones by taking insulin and fluids regularly. Extra insulin is the key which helps switch off the ketone-producing mechanism in the body. The more ketones we have the more insulin we require. The dose may need to be increased if there is a suboptimal response.

Blood Ketone level	Action required
< 0.6 mmol/l	Okay and no action needed
0.6-1.5 mmol/l	This is a warning sign and correction via pen and more frequent monitoring is needed.

| > 1.5 mmol/l | Take quick action and seek urgent medical help. |

3.5 Diabetic ketoacidosis (DKA) and illness

DKA can result from insufficient insulin or during illness. During illness our body becomes more resistant to insulin, so when your patient is ill he/she may require additional insulin. Sickness can also cause stress hormones release, and these can cause glucose levels to raise more.

Management of diabetes during illness:

Patients with diabetes need extra insulin when they are unwell and will need even more if blood ketones are present.

Consider problems with insulin delivery. Remember that the patient has no long-acting insulin; they are dependent on fast-acting insulin only, which, after two to three hours, will see BG levels rapidly rise if delivery stops or the needle comes out.

1. Check for possible needle misplacement or dislodgement.
2. Check for air bubbles in the tube.
3. Remember, problems are likely to occur quickly if your patient has missed insulin or his diabetes is poorly controlled with high HbA1c.
4. Consider switching to a pen and cartridge insulin.
5. Check for ketones more frequently.
6. If they have had something to eat in the last 1-2 hours, re-check in one hour as they may not have taken enough insulin for the amount they ate, or a different type of bolus may have worked better for the type or quantity of food they ate.
7. It is recommended that your patient's blood is tested for ketones if their blood glucose levels are over 14 mmol/l (>250mg/dl). Ask them to take their usual correction dose but be aware this may need to be increased in the presence of ketones and give them plenty of water or sugar-free fluid.
8. If they do not want to eat, offer sweetened fluid and give an insulin bolus accordingly.
9. Identify the cause of high blood glucose, starting with infusion set change, (change the infusion set if in any doubt) check pump settings and seek help/treatment as necessary.
10. Blood glucose and ketones need to be tested every one to two hours and repeat the correction dose until blood ketones start to clear. Most people

need to increase their usual correction dose when ketones are present. Give the correction dose by pen if no response and ketones are present.
11. Consider pre-setting an illness basal pattern rate.
12. Correct high blood glucose levels with the usual correction ratio providing the child is ketone free. If blood glucose levels are allowed to get out of hand, DKA can occur very quickly.
13. Child should not exercise if ketones are high and the healthcare team should be contacted if high blood glucose levels and ketones persist and/or vomiting starts.
14. Aggressive management of blood glucose levels is necessary at times of illness.
15. If their blood glucose levels are very high (even in the absence of ketones) you may find the usual correction dose may not be enough.
16. In the presence of ketones, give insulin by pen until back under control. You will need more insulin than usual. Some adults and teenagers need to double their usual correction dose.
17. Use the temporary basal rate to increase in 20% steps and check blood glucose levels every one to two hours to see if this needs to be repeated.
18. You may need to increase the "max basal rate" for the duration of the illness. Don't forget to reduce it once your patient is better.
19. Once blood glucose levels are less than 10mmol/l (<180 mg/dl), start to gradually reduce the insulin in 20% steps, provided that the result was not preceded by the administration of a correction dose within the last two hours.

3.6 Testing and adjusting basal rate

Blood glucose levels are affected by many variables including:
1. Food
2. Activity
3. Basal insulin
4. Bolus insulin – mealtime and correction boluses
5. Other factors, such as illness, stress, medications, growth and other hormones.

In the absence of food, exercise and mealtime/bolus insulin, basal insulin should hold the blood sugar steady.

Why is basal rate testing important?
1- Having the right basal rate keeps blood sugars in the right range overnight and between meals.
2- If basal rate is too low, blood sugar could go too high.

3- If basal rate is too high, blood sugar could go low.
4- Testing basal rate can help to find the right basal rates for your patients.

Basal rate testing is a process that examines the insulin pump basal rate, while trying to eliminate or minimize the influence of other factors. Testing should not be performed during an illness or onset of menses, following hypoglycaemia, or if the blood sugar is greater than 250 mg/dl at the beginning of the test. Basal rates should be checked every six to eight weeks, every school holiday and before Ramadan for those fasting to ensure your patient's programmed basal rate is meeting their body's requirement for the background supply of insulin. Insulin dose will need to be gradually increased in children as they grow and develop, and this becomes more important during growth spurts.

The simplest way to test the basal rate is to divide the day into several time windows, where people are following a normal routine with no strenuous activity preceding or during the period of testing and not taking any carbohydrates (ideally fasting for the entire period). This allows normal state basal requirements to be determined. An example of a protocol is given below. Basal rate testing can be performed and repeated as often as required. Timings can be varied and test periods can be focused on problem times.

How to test basal rate

1- Fast (no CHO) for a period of 2-6 hours depending on age and ability to fast. This may not be possible for children younger than six. Therefore, you may delay eating for as long as possible. Give last CHO two hours before starting to fast and try to avoid low glycaemic index foods. Your patient should not eat any snacks during the fast period (they can drink water). For small children where you can't omit a meal, delay it as long as you can or give a standard meal with a known amount of CHO and high GI (e.g. toast).
2- Blood glucose level should stay within their targets, if their basal rate is appropriate for them.
3- We need to consider when they last had a bolus, ate some food and what it was they ate, as these could still be affecting their blood glucose. Slowly-absorbed food may have an effect on blood sugar for up to 6 hours.
4- Give normal insulin bolus with last meal, use current basal rates and check blood glucose level every one to two hours during the fast.
5- Avoid testing during illness, following hypoglycaemia or after exercise (i.e. no hypoglycaemia or strenuous activity in the last 24 hours). Test overnight basal first, then breakfast until lunch, lunch until evening meal, and lastly evening meal until bed. It is best not to test these all on the same day.

6- Abandon the test if hypo (blood glucose under 4 mmol/l / 72 mg/dl) or hyperglycaemia occurs (blood glucose over 14 mmol/l / 250 mg/dl) and treat accordingly.
7- Record blood glucose, basal rate, carbohydrate content of food before and any other variables.
8- Once complete, you can change your patient's basal rate if needed.

Is it basal or bolus?

Identifying the contribution of basal and bolus insulin to recurrent hyper- and hypoglycaemia can be difficult. Continuous glucose monitoring can suggest mismatch between insulin and food. Therefore, basal rate testing may identify issues with the basal rates. Don't make more than one change at a time as multiple changes can be confusing. Review the impact of your changes over several days.

Consider the basal amount or timing needs adjustments for:
1. Blood glucose variations (low or high) during the night or before breakfast.
2. Low or high glucose if a meal is skipped or delayed.

Consider the bolus adjustments (including the ICR and ISF) for:
1. High or low glucose within 4 h of a bolus or meal.
2. Hypoglycaemia following a correction insulin bolus.

Basal Insulin Testing requirements:

1- No consumption of any calories during the basal test, unless your blood glucose drops low. The meal/snack preceding the basal test should be low in fat. Patient can have water, diet beverages and other non-caloric foods during the test.
2- Monitor blood glucose levels every 1-2 hours during daytime tests and every 2-3 hours during overnight tests
3- No bolus during the test, unless your blood glucose is above 250.
4- Do not suspend pump.
5- Do not have a temporary basal rate running.
6- Do not disconnect from the pump.
7- Do not change your tubing, cartridge or infusion set during the test.
8- No hypoglycemic episodes for at least 6 hours preceding the basal test.
9- No steroid medications being used.
10- No illnesses during the testing (fever, infection, virus).
11- Avoid testing basal rates within two days of starting a menstrual cycle.
12- Allow basal insulin to be delivered uninterrupted
13- Maintain low-moderate activity level

Basal testing can be done in many ways as shown in Table 3.4.

Table 3.4

A- Overnight basal testing 22:00-06:00	B- Morning basal testing 06:00-12:00	C- Afternoon basal testing 12:00-18:00	D- Evening basal testing 18:00-22:00
1-Basal testing period between 22:00 and 06:00. 2- Evening meal before 19:00, after which no further food (ensure evening meal is easy to CHO count to avoid errors in CHO counting, which may impact testing period). 3- Test blood glucose at 22:00, 00:00, 03:00 and 06:00. 4-Breakfast and bolus at 06:00.	1- Basal testing period between 06:00 and 12:00. 2- Proceed only if fasting glucose in target. 3- Test blood glucose at 06:00, 08:00, 10:00 and 12:00. 4-Lunch and bolus at 12:00.	1- Basal testing period between 12:00 and 18:00. 2- Proceed only if pre-lunch glucose in target and omit lunch. 3- Test blood glucose at 12:00, 14:00, 16:00 and 18:00. 4- Usual dinner and bolus at 18:00.	1- Basal testing period between 18:00 and 22:00. 2- Proceed only if pre-dinner glucose in target and omit dinner. 3- Test blood glucose at 18:00, 20:00 and 22:00. 4- Evening meal and bolus at 22:00.
Basal rates can be assessed using continuous glucose monitoring (CGM) to record glucose values during fasting or low carbohydrate intake. This can be achieved using retrospective continuous glucose monitoring or real-time monitoring. In the event of hypoglycaemic or hyperglycaemic symptoms, the pump users should test their capillary blood glucose and treat accordingly.			

Interpretation and adjusting insulin during basal testing

To ensure appropriate interpretation of continuous glucose monitoring, normal basal rates should be used during the period of monitoring and a recording sheet should be completed, including meals, mealtime, capillary blood glucose and insulin doses. Also record basal rates, bolus and correction bolus.

1. When the blood glucose does not remain stable within +/- 2 mmol/l, adjustments of the basal rate is recommended. Adjust if blood glucose varies (increases or decreases) by 2 mmol/L or 35 mg/dl during a 4 hour period. Some children need more insulin with breakfast, due to the effects of the dawn phenomenon.
2. Adjust basal rate by 0.025–0.1 unit/h (10–20% increase or decrease) at a time depending on age, sensitivity and total daily dose. Repeat on another day to see if it is now correct.

3. Make appropriate adjustment 1–2 h before blood glucose change.

3.7 Testing and adjusting insulin to carbohydrate ratio

When the basal rate is tested and corrected, looking for problems in the bolus becomes more straightforward. When analysing pump data, glucose excursions 2–4 h after a bolus can be addressed if other factors are excluded. The meals at the end of the basal tests provide a useful picture of the ICR if a 2-h and 4-h blood glucose test is undertaken.

If ICR is right for your patient, their blood glucose level should be no more than 2 mmol/l (or 35 mg/dl) higher or lower than their pre-meal blood glucose level 2-4 hours after eating. For example, if their blood glucose is 6 mmol/l before breakfast and < 8 mmol/l two hours later, the ratio is correct.

Possible problems with glucose after bolus insulin are summarised in Table 3.5.

Table 3.5 Causes for hyper and hypoglycaemia after insulin bolus

1- Bolus calculation
Check log book/food diaries for possible errors.
Use bolus calculator to minimise errors.
2- Carbohydrate counting
Check in clinic with visual aids/prompts.
Smartphone pictures or food diaries can help.
3- ICR
Assess using simple/easy ways to count meals.
Remember ICR can vary during different times of the day.
4- ISF
Look for impact of correction doses on glucose when other variables are not changing.
5- Other factors as discussed above

3.8 Continuous glucose monitoring (CGM)

When moving onto the pump it becomes even more important to monitor blood glucose. CGM blood glucose meters and downloads from the pump should be offered to your patients to maximise the benefits of the pump.

In children without diabetes, background insulin secretion varies depending on the time of day and night. This is particularly important in teenagers when they are going through a growth spurt. The insulin pump gives you the opportunity to mimic this. To help you get it right, it is important to download your meter and pump readings to see what changes you need to make.

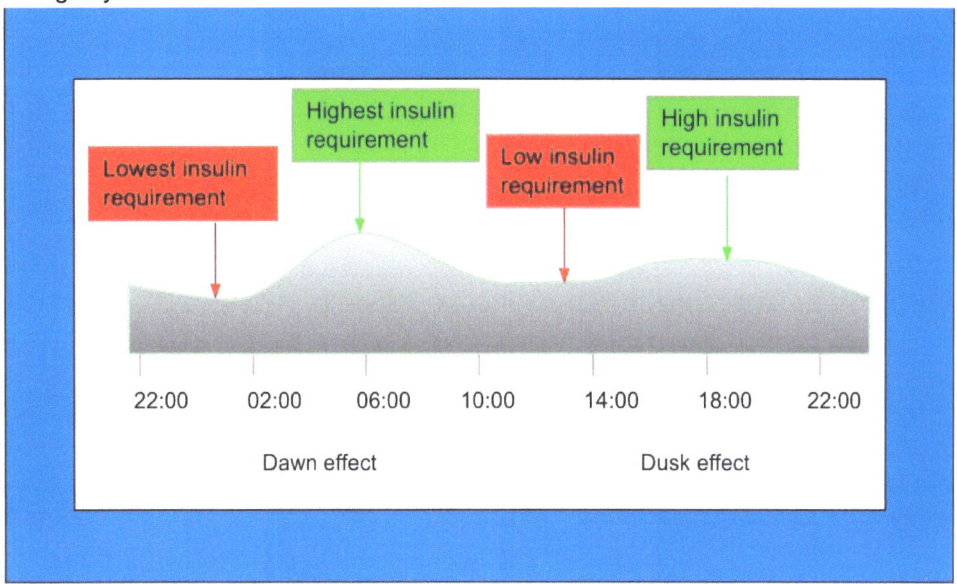

Figure 3.1 Dawn and Dusk phenomenon

Dawn phenomenon

Sometimes called the dawn effect, the dawn phenomenon is an early-morning (usually between 2am and 8am) hyperglycaemic excursion relevant to people with diabetes. It is different from chronic Somogyi rebound in that it is not preceded by nocturnal hypoglycaemia. It is caused by counter-regulatory hormones (such as adrenaline, growth hormone and cortisol) being secreted prior to waking.

Dawn phenomenon is difficult to manage with MDI regimens. An insulin pump can be effective in managing the dawn effect without causing hypoglycaemia. This is achieved by allowing increased insulin to be delivered during the early hours of the morning.

Continuous subcutaneous insulin infusion (insulin pump) helps to improve the overnight glucose profile due to the dawn phenomenon. It is advised to increase basal rates by 20-30%) from 02:00 to 06:00am. ICR at breakfast should be increased.

In children frequent overnight testing can be very inconvenient; however, CGM provides a convenient way to assess and improve overnight glycaemic control and often reveals issues not noted previously.

Dusk phenomenon

The dusk phenomenon is a spontaneous and transient pre-dinner hyperglycaemia. It is not as well-known as the dawn effect and it is objective in some children with diabetes. The dusk phenomenon in diabetic patients is common but often ignored by doctors. Awareness of the dusk phenomenon has important clinical significance because it can affect blood glucose control between post-dinner and pre-bed. It can be controlled by increasing insulin dosage before dinner by insulin pump.

Continuous glucose monitors

Continuous glucose monitors (CGM) is an advanced way to check glucose readings in real-time or monitor glucose readings over a period of time. It provides information about glucose concentration in the interstitial fluid, which is present in under the skin.
A CGM system consists of three parts: a glucose sensor (Fig. 3.2), a transmitter and a receiver or a monitor that displays the glucose information. The monitor connects either wirelessly, via a wireless transmitter attached to the sensor, or by a cable to the sensor. New generations of CGM devices can transmit glucose data to compatible mobile phones.

The continuous glucose sensor is inserted via a small cannula under the skin and is attached to a transmitter. The sensor communicates to a receiver and can display real-time glucose. To ensure accuracy the sensor data needs to be calibrated to capillary blood glucose, typically, one to three times per day, depending on manufacturer. However, some new generations of CGM do not require calibration.

CGM sensors measure the glucose concentration every 5 minutes. They report interstitial glucose levels between around 2 and 22 mmol/L (36- 400 mg/dl). Values above or below this range cannot be reported. The sensors should be changed typically every 6-7 days, depending on manufacturer.
Some CGM models can send information right away to a second person's Smartphone—perhaps a parent or caregiver. For example, if a child's glucose drops dangerously low at school or overnight, the CGM could be set to alert a parent at home.

Table 3.6 shows the differences between real-time and retrospective continuous glucose monitoring. Retrospective CGM requires no input from your patient during use and it is easy to use. It requires calibration with capillary blood glucose values, but this is done after the monitoring period.

A handheld monitor system displays up to 8 hours of retrospective continuous glucose monitoring data, along with a trend arrow and a glucose value, when the monitor is waved close to a subcutaneous glucose sensor.

In contrast to real-time CGM, the intermittent CGM system does not provide alarms for high or low glucose. Stored retrospective data can be downloaded and visualised. The sensor is used for 14 days and is non-adjunctive, which means that the reported glucose values do not require verification with capillary blood glucose before diabetes treatment decisions are made.

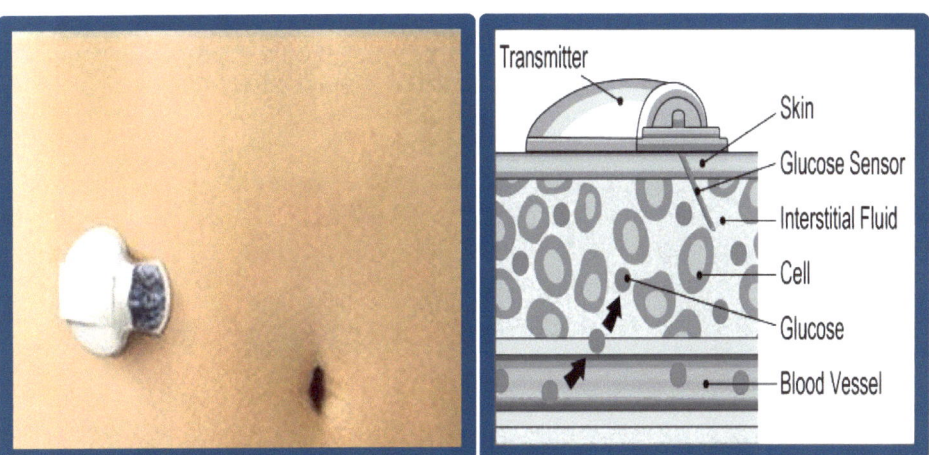

Figure 3.2 Continuous glucose monitoring (CGM) device.

Why is CGM important in diabetes?

1- CGM replaces the finger stick picture.

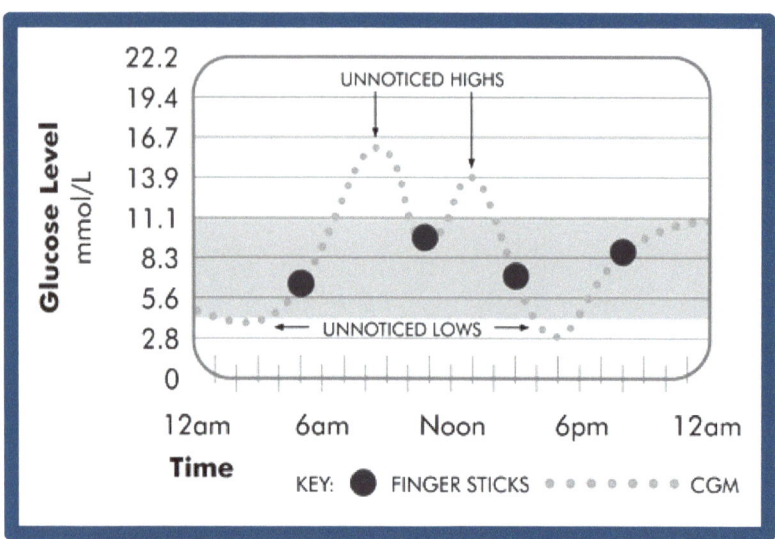

Figure 3.3 Complete picture

2- The use of alerts allows early intervention to reduce the severity and duration of highs and lows.
3- CGM shows frequency, magnitude and duration of excursions.
4- It reflects glucose variability and hypoglycaemia.
5- Allows integration with pumps.
6- Data can be analysed.

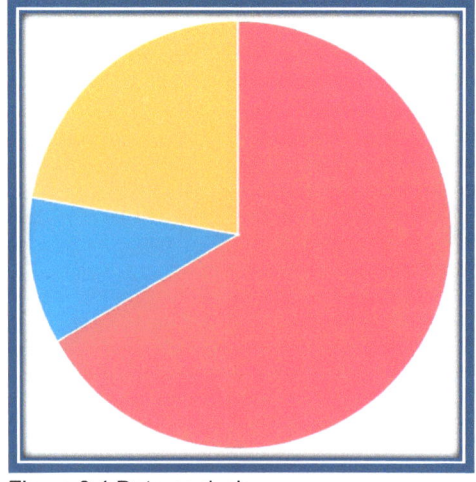

65% within target range
22% above target range
13% below target range

Figure 3.4 Data analysis

60

Possible problems with glucose sensing

1. Cost
2. Accuracy
3. Alarm fatigue
4. Dislodgment (more frequent in small children)
5. Skin irritation and infection (rare)
6. Accurate calibration is needed as per careful instructions and finger prick testing. If calibration is not done, readings will be meaningless
7. There is an approximate 15 to 20 minute delay when comparing blood glucose levels and glucose levels under the skin. It is therefore best at picking up trends and will not necessarily pick up rapid hypos. When you get unexpected or doubtful readings, check blood glucose.
8. The needle cannot be left in place for more than six days and should be taken out if the area looks red and inflamed.

Advise your patients/parents:

1. To ensure the date and time is correct on all meters (remember to check after battery changes).
2. To bring all meters to be downloaded to appointments, including the one used at school.
3. To remember clock changes in autumn and spring.

Meter downloading can be done at home and data can be accessed by the healthcare team to review the results.

Table 3.6 Types of CGM (classification depends on purpose of use).

	Real time	Retrospective analysis (professional, masked)
Intended user	Patient	Healthcare professionals, patient
Patient education	Continuous and immediate	Episodic and retrospective
Purpose	Immediate changes in behaviour, such as diet, medications, insulin dosage, physical activity. Patient education	To estimate quality of glycaemic control, magnitude of glycaemic variability, times of day with highest risks of hypo- and hyperglycaemia.

	needed regarding effects of diet, exercise, medications, insulin on glucose levels, variability and patterns.	Identification of patterns that can be subsequently used to make long-term changes in diet, medications, insulin and physical activity, if patterns are stable over days.
Real-time display of results	Display for glucose, rate of change of glucose, alerts/alarms, graphical display is immediately available. Data from real-time systems can also be analysed retrospectively.	Not available. However, this approach is useful when immediate behaviour change is not required (e.g. for some clinical trials).

Blood glucose versus interstitial fluid glucose

Continuous glucose monitoring may reduce the frequency of tests needed in some cases, but it is not a replacement for capillary blood glucose monitoring. They also can be a very powerful tool for management, education and support.

Glucose concentration in the interstitial fluid is dependent on blood flow, rate of glucose change in the blood and the metabolic rate. Trends in interstitial fluid glucose represent changes in blood glucose concentrations but peak glucose concentrations in interstitial fluid lag behind changes in blood glucose concentration by around 10-15 min. CGM users should ideally calibrate when glucose is as stable as possible to optimize the sensor accuracy. This will often be before bed and first thing in the morning. Avoid calibrating CGM devices at times of rapid glucose change, e.g. following meals or exercise.

Calibration is to ensure the continuous glucose monitor is as accurate as possible. The closer the sensor reading to the blood glucose meter reading, the better the accuracy. Calibration during a rapid change in glucose will lead to a large difference between blood and interstitial fluid glucose.

Why to use CGM

CGM devices are used to assess glucose profiles in children with consistent glucose problems on insulin therapy. It has benefits in combination with intensive insulin therapy. Continuous glucose monitoring is useful in guiding insulin adjustments for people with type 1 diabetes using insulin pump therapy or multiple dose insulin injection regimens. It also results in reduction in HbA_{1c} after continuous use, and, hence, reduction in long-term diabetes complications, such as retinopathy, nephropathy and neuropathy.

CGM can identify and prevent unwanted periods of hyperglycaemia and hypoglycaemia, enhancing diabetes management and reduction of glucose variability.

To benefit from CGM, children with diabetes or their caregivers should be encouraged to participate in their diabetes care and, in particular, act on the results of the CGM. Sometimes, recording of events (such as mealtimes, exercise, stress and hypoglycaemic symptoms) can be helpful.

Indications for use:

Continuous monitoring may be particularly useful in CSII where the ability to alter basal rates can be exploited.

1. Consistent disparity between capillary blood glucose self-monitoring results and HbA_{1c}.
2. Haemoglobinopathy affecting red cell life span.
3. Impaired hypoglycaemia awareness (or hypoglycaemia unawareness), recurrent and disabling hypoglycaemia or debilitating fear of hypoglycaemia.
4. Poor glycaemic control, despite intensive treatment and appropriate self-management.
5. During activity and exercise to monitor blood glucose level
6. Suspected dawn phenomenon.
7. To evaluate the effect of a specific change in therapy.
8. During illness.
9. In people who exercise (to minimize hypoglycaemia).
10. In children with normal glucose tolerance (to provide additional information to usual investigation protocols).
11. In the investigation of insulin secreting tumours (insulinomas).
12. For type 2 diabetes.

According to National Institute of Clinical Excellency (NICE), CGM is recommended for children with type 1 diabetes treated with pumps or multiple daily injections (MDI) in the following settings:

1. Patient is keen to use it at least 70% of time with required calibrations.
2. Fear of hypoglycaemia.
3. Hypoglycaemia unawareness.
4. Disabling hypoglycaemia, especially at night.
5. Two episodes per week of asymptomatic hypoglycaemia leading to problems with daily activities.
6. More than one episode a year of severe hypoglycaemia that has no obvious/preventable cause.

Intermittent CGM is also recommended for retrospective diagnostics, especially in the following circumstances: nocturnal hypoglycaemia, dawn phenomenon, postprandial hyperglycaemia, and changes to diabetes regimen.

Contraindications

There are no specific contraindications to CGM. However, continuous monitoring should not be undertaken in the following conditions:

1- Peripheral circulatory failure and severe dehydration. These conditions cause peripheral shutdown, which can cause artificially low readings.
2- Some renal dialysis treatments: children undergoing peritoneal dialysis, as maltose (a disaccharide of two glucose molecules) used by the enzyme electrode may affect the readings.
3- Hyperlipidaemia: cholesterol levels above 12 mmol/L may lead to artificially raised capillary blood glucose readings
4- Haematocrit values above 55% may lead to inaccurate levels if the blood glucose level is more than 11mol/L (198mg/dl)
5- Generalised skin infection, rash or eczema.

Points to consider when inserting CGM sensors

To ensure accuracy and reduce interference, sensors are usually inserted in the abdomen (Figure 3.2), but other sites, such as the upper outer buttock or arm can be used. We also need to consider the following points:

1- Insert sensor 5 cm away from an insulin pump infusion cannula and 5-7 cm from a syringe or insulin pen injection site. Sensors may be a little painful when first inserted but are flexible and it is unusual to experience significant discomfort while using them. There is low risk of bleeding and infection.
2- Insert 3-5 cm away from any recent sensor insertion sites.
3- Insert 3-5 cm away from the umbilicus.

4- Avoid areas where there is regular bending or the risk of chaffing from clothing, such as waistbands to reduce the risk of dislodgement or damage, both of which can affect the quality of data collected.
5- Avoid areas with lipohypertrophy, marks, stretch scars or hardened tissue.
6- Sensors are secured with dressings. Be vigilant of any signs of skin infection or bleeding and gauge whether the sensor is dislodged.
7- Most sensors and transmitters are water-resistant, so users are able to shower, bathe or swim while the continuous monitor is in situ.

Continuous glucose monitoring (CGM) is helpful in the self-management of diabetes and real-time CGM can help children with type 1 diabetes achieve a reduction in HbA_{1c} and /or reduced frequency and severity of hypoglycaemia. Children with diabetes using real-time CGM are most likely to achieve these goals if they are able to wear a sensor continuously at least 70% of the time. Appropriate support by expert healthcare professionals is required to ensure calibrations are done when glucose levels are likely to be stable. Use the trend arrow rather than the absolute value to make treatment decisions.

To minimize alarm fatigue, patients need to set personalized alarm thresholds and review them periodically.

Patients should not ignore any symptoms of hypo- and hyperglycaemia, regardless of the CGM readings.

Alarm Feature

The monitors can be set to alarm when the glucose is outside certain ranges (i.e. during hypo- and hyperglycaemia) and when the rate of change of glucose is very steep. It can be set to alarm before low, at low, before high and at high levels. Ensure alarms are set appropriately to avoid alarm fatigue. Careful calibration of the sensor will ensure that the sensor signal is optimal and will maximise the likelihood of the alarms being correct. Healthcare support of management of hypo- and hyperglycaemia will empower children and carers to take the appropriate action.

Initial alarms may be set wide apart (e.g. at 70 mg/dl and 250 mg/dl) to minimise the frequency of alarms until the child/carer is comfortable with the frequency of alarms. Then can be moved closer to the target range gradually and can be set earlier than the target to take early action and prevent hypoglycaemia. This can be done to prevent hyperglycaemia if postprandial hyperglycaemia is the problem. Setting earlier alarms may allow for an insulin correction bolus before significant hyperglycaemia occurs. Over time, this may have an effect on hypoglycaemia awareness. Different alarm thresholds can be set for different times in some CGM devices. One of the biggest barriers to using real-time CGM is alarm fatigue, therefore minimising the number of alarms, especially at night, can also help to prevent alarm fatigue.

Another useful feature on real-time continuous glucose monitors is the snooze feature. It notifies the pump user if a high or low glucose state has not changed after a pre-set time. Hence, it allows time to treat hypo- or hyperglycaemia but, if the insulin correction or carbohydrate was insufficient, the device will alarm after a pre-set number of minutes or hours. The snooze time can be set at any time but should be lower (10-20 min) for the hypoglycaemia alarm as treatment of hypoglycaemia should take effect rapidly. A longer snooze time can be used for the hyperglycaemia alarm (2-3 hrs).

To take appropriate action before high or low targets are reached, a predictive alert is another feature of CGM that warns us if glucose levels are predicted to become high or low or if there is a sharp upward or downward trend.

In some devices the rate of change threshold can also be programmed (e.g. 5mg/dl/min). In this case the CGM will alarm if the rise or fall in glucose is greater than the rate of change threshold, regardless of the absolute glucose value. When this feature is set correctly, it can be very useful in warning ahead of low or high sugars.

Remember that capillary blood glucose monitoring devices may be up to 15% different from a reference a blood glucose measurement. The absolute glucose value displayed on the CGM may be inaccurate, with values up to 9-13% different from capillary blood. This means the value displayed by CGM is a guide only. However, the trend arrow displays the direction and velocity of glucose rate of change. For example, if the glucose is 10.0 mmol/L (180mg/dl) two hours after a meal and the trend arrow indicates a rapid increase in glucose, this may suggest a problem with the insulin pump, an insufficient mealtime bolus or delayed absorption of food, and an additional bolus might be considered. But, if the glucose is 9.0 mmol/L (162mg/dl) two hours after a meal and is falling, this may be the end of a mealtime peak and watching the glucose fall to target may be the appropriate action. In this case, the trend arrow helps with the treatment decision and the absolute glucose value could be anywhere between 7 and 12 mmol/L.

Stable	→
Falling slowly	↘

Falling quickly	↓
Falling rapidly	↓↓
Raising slowly	↗
Raising quickly	↑
Raising rapidly	↑↑

Figure 3.6 Trend arrow displaying direction and value of glucose change.

Sensor-augmented pump therapy (figure 1.5)

Sensor-augmented pump therapy is a combination of three main components: insulin pump, continuous glucose monitoring (CGM) system and therapy management software. This system incorporates innovative CGM features like predictive alerts to prevent dangerous hypo or hyperglycaemic glucose events.

The insulin pump acts as the receiver of the CGM data sent wirelessly from the sensor by the transmitter. As with real-time CGM, an absolute interstitial fluid glucose concentration is reported, along with a trace of the preceding hours and a trend arrow.

The pump is also able to switch off insulin infusion in response to hypoglycaemia or even in advance of predicted hypoglycaemia. The insulin infusion can be suspended for either a fixed time (of up to 2 hours) or until the glucose rises above a threshold.

This feature allows insulin delivery to be suspended automatically for up to two hours when the continuous glucose monitor detects that the glucose level has fallen and there is a risk of hypoglycaemia. The ability to suspend insulin reduces the magnitude and frequency of hypoglycaemia overnight. Sensor-augmented pumps are an advance from standard insulin pumps but are not yet perfected to the point where insulin can be automatically dispensed based on the glucose reading. However, it is the first step towards a closed loop insulin delivery system ('artificial pancreas').

An artificial pancreas is a device that closely mimics the glucose-regulating function of a healthy pancreas. It not only monitors glucose levels in the body but also automatically adjusts the delivery of insulin to reduce hyperglycaemia and minimise the incidence of hypoglycaemia with little or no input from the patient. Patients are advised to always confirm their sensor glucose reading using their BG meter, and follow the instructions of your healthcare professional to treat low glucose.

Currently available artificial devices may not be safe for use in small children under the age of 7 because of the way that the system is designed and the daily insulin requirements of at least 8 units per day.

3.8 Meter/pump downloads, interpretation of blood glucose readings and decision making

All insulin pumps have an upload system and most of them allow data to be analysed and displayed in formats that are easy to understand and interpret. It also allows visualization of basal, bolus, food, carbohydrate counting, behavioural patterns, as well as other very useful data during clinic visits or remotely. Some smartphone apps allow data entry and logging. Patients can upload their data and email it to healthcare professionals to obtain periodic advice via e-mail or telephone.

All meters have the facility to download blood glucose readings so that the healthcare team, patients and parents can analyse and interpret them. It is important to take time each week to review your patient's glucose results and see if changes are required.

If you can get the initial basal rate, ICR and ISF settings correct at the beginning it will lead to good control and make it easier to review at regular intervals and keep good control. Before taking action or making any major changes, remember to confirm values obtained from real-time continuous monitors using capillary blood glucose measurement, particularly in the absence of symptoms.

Due to the limited accuracy of CGMs, particularly in the hypoglycaemic range, glycaemic excursion and trends data are key elements to obtain from CGM. Data obtained from CGM are best interpreted with other information, including meals, exercise, insulin administered and hypoglycaemic symptoms. Retrospective glucose monitoring should be analysed and the impact of the monitoring period should be assessed during the clinic visit considering other related factors.

It is important to have the pump and/or meters data downloaded before or during the clinic visit, prior to consultation, as this helps you make appropriate decisions. This usually requires having relevant software and additional time. Pump users may be able to upload their own data before visits and/or bring printouts with them.

How to interpret CGM – a suggested approach

Practice and familiarity with the way the data is presented helps in quick reviewing and decision-making. You need a systematic and easy approach to interpret and extract useful information. The approach below is one you may consider:

Patient details and basic information:
Ensure you are looking at your patient's data, check child's name, date of birth, hospital number, type of diabetes, treatment regimen, how many days was the sensor worn for; whether it is a retrospective or real-time trace and what the indication was for CGM.

Other basic information you should check are:
- a- Pump programmes: basal profiles, total daily dose, ICR and ISF. Basal:bolus ratio, although it is difficult to make generalizations, a ratio of 40:60 is typical for children. The basal may be lower if the child is very active. Large deviations from this ratio may prompt consideration of whether the correct basal or bolus doses are being used.
- b- Average testing, at least 4–6 times a day are expected with pumps.
- c- Percentages (high and low) can give a glimpse of how much time is being spent outside the desired range and in hypoglycaemia. This will be overrepresented if people test more when they 'feel' high or low.
- d- Average carbohydrate intake: usually around 200 g/day, but varies.
- e- Set changes: every 2–3 days.

Ensure CGM data are sufficient
CGM software provides reports with the data presented in different ways. Each datum consists of more than one report and it is important to look at each report as they usually offer different information. Review overall trace to ensure that the information is robust enough to make any treatment decisions. Any reports with missing sections of data with changes that do not correlate with the diary or symptoms should be reviewed with caution. One frequent example is a period of time where the sensor glucose is much higher or lower than the capillary value.

Most sensors record glucose every 5 minutes, this means 288 values in a complete 24-hour period. Fewer than 288 values suggest missing data and it is important to identify the cause.

Mean absolute difference (MAD %)

MAD % is available on some CGM reports as a percentage or 'mean absolute relative difference' (MARD). The MAD% gives an idea of sensor accuracy. In most studies, the MAD% for sensors is between 10% and 15%, suggesting that the sensor glucose is within 15% of the capillary blood glucose. For example, a reported sensor glucose of 9 mmol/L (180 mg/dl) is equivalent to capillary blood glucose between 7.5 and 10.5 mmol/l (117- 190 mg/dl).

Daily overlay view (modal day view)

Daily overlay view (also known as modal day view) is the most popular way of reviewing CGM traces. It shows each day of the monitoring period drawn on top of each other (usually in different colours), showing patterns of glucose change over several days or weeks, as shown in Figure 3.8.

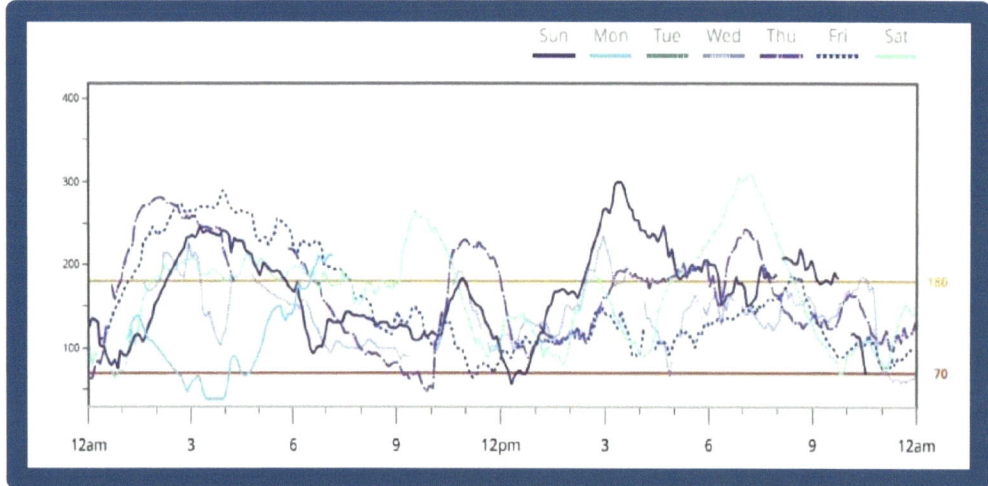

Figure 3.8 Daily overlay view

How to interpret the daily overlay

- a- Determine if there is any clear pattern repeated on each day or through a part of each day.
- b- Prioritize your targets: look at hypos before hyperglycaemia, look at night time pattern before daytime patterns and more frequent abnormalities than single and isolated abnormalities.

c- Consider overnight, first three hours post meals, then three hours or more post meals. Breaking the 24 hrs up into sections of the day allows the identification of trends; for example, times where there are frequent high or low glucose excursions and periods of the day where the same glucose changes occur.
d- Look for any repeated hypoglycaemia, particularly overnight, before meals and after exercise.
e- Look for any recurrent hyperglycaemia (particularly after meals) and patterns of upsloping or downsloping trends.
f- Ignore outliers or extreme isolated hyperglycaemia or hypoglycaemia episodes. (Exceptions and outliers will be discussed later – step 10).
g- Look at overnight, fasting, during and after exercise, and before and after meals. (Use the activity and food diary to confirm and support the timings.)
h- Remember to trace changes back, as glucose effects of exercise in diabetes may occur several hours later or even the next day.
i- As a general rule, steep gradient upsloping trends reflect food intake and gradual upsloping may be due to inadequate basal insulin, stress or small snacks.
j- Steep gradient downsloping trends reflect insulin action on glucose and gradual downsloping may be related to activity, increased basal insulin or insulin taken with meal.

Daily summaries

Are there excessive increases or decreases? Are these changes related to exercise, school, snacks or other lifestyle events?

The data summary or the statistics summary is another area to look at. Data include the number of glucose values, mean sensor glucose, highest value, lowest value, mean capillary blood glucose, standard deviation (SD) and the percentage of time spent in hypoglycaemia, hyperglycaemia and target as shown below.
These values are usually given each day for overall monitoring and, where needed, target ranges can be personalised.

The lowest and highest values give the range of glucose, but it should be remembered that all sensors have a high and low limit of detection. Where the high or low sensor glucose ranges are the same as the limit of detection of the sensor, the actual glucose may have risen higher or fallen lower.

The mean sensor glucose is the average of all glucose values and the mean capillary blood glucose is the average of the calibration glucose results. These might be very different from each other, depending on the glucose excursions seen in the CGM trace. The SD of the sensor glucose is a measure of spread of glucose values and is an indicator of glucose variability. The percentage time spent in hypoglycaemia, target and hyperglycaemia gives an idea of overall glucose patterns.

Consider the pattern (trend)

Find a pattern of glucose readings over the last days or weeks. See if this pattern follows a specific event, e.g. a specific meal, exercise or certain food. This relies on looking at the pooled average glucose data and spotting obvious trends. Looking at a large amount of data graphically provides a much more easy and powerful way of picking up a trend than looking at diaries. You notice the difference if your patients did not bring his meters or you can't download the data from the pump due to internet issues. Downloaded data also allows visualization of glucose patterns against basal, bolus and meal patterns to make adjustments to therapy. When looking to pick up trends, it is useful to break up the day into the following windows:
- a- overnight period
- b- breakfast to lunch
- c- lunch to dinner
- d- dinner to bedtime.

Trends to look out for:

- a- Overnight glucose control
- b- Hypoglycaemia (time/preceding activity/bolus)
- c- Glucose control after hypoglycaemia (reflects correct correction ratio)
- d- Hyperglycaemia
- e- Glucose control after hyperglycaemia (reflects correct correction ratio)
- f- Pre-meal glucose control
- g- Glucose control after meal
- h- Glucose control after exercise.

Remove distractions

If no patterns are identified using earlier steps, using a piece of paper, block out 4-10 mmol/l(72-180mg/dl) on the daily overlay view to assess where the hypo- and hyperglycaemic excursions are occurring. This is useful to demonstrate the number and pattern of excursions very clearly and examine outliers or isolated lows and highs. Tracing excursions back identifies the cause. Masking also helps you to focus and concentrate more by reducing unnecessary distractions.

Details (day-by-day view)

Looking at this view allows you to view each day individually and each glucose excursion or event can be correlated with the diary and the glucose effects of specific activities or foods. It also allows you to notice the difference between weekdays and weekends, changes during periods of stress, school days and changes over the menstrual cycle.

This view assesses overnight glucose control, patterns of hypoglycaemia, effects of correction doses and patterns of rebound hyperglycaemia. It also assesses post-hypoglycaemia treatment, pre- and postprandial glucose control and effects of lifestyle, exercise and stress.

Identify problems

Is it high BG, low BG, fluctuation or dawn phenomenon? What time and how often does the problem occur?

Prioritise problem and identify the possible causes

If you have no pattern and glucose values are up and down with many hypos and hyperglycaemias, we need to prioritise the problems based on their significance and the harm they can cause to children and their families.

    a- Night-time lows
    b- Daytime lows
    c- Night-time highs
    d- Daytime highs

Hypoglycaemia at night is more dangerous than during the day as it can go unnoticed, leading to fits or making the child tired the next day.

Exceptions / outliers

These are extreme highs and lows, which affect the child most. They are often reflective of issues concerning:

    a- Correction of hyperglycaemia (overcorrection or stacking leading to hypoglycaemia)
    b- Errors in carbohydrate counting
    c- Missed or miscalculated boluses
    d- Set change problems (delayed set change may lead to high blood glucose levels)
    e- Unanticipated activity or stresses.

Taking a detailed and focused history from your patients and their families can identify the reasons for these outliers.

Provide potential solutions

Avoid making more than two changes in one session. However, this depends on many factors, including patient age, availability of healthcare team and parents'/carers' sensibility and understanding.

3.9 Using CGM to manage difficult diabetes situations

Hypoglycaemia unawareness

Some children with hypoglycaemia unawareness do not have symptoms associated with low glucose levels and do not mount a counter-regulatory response to hypoglycaemia, which leaves them exposed to frequent hypoglycaemia and for prolonged periods. The risk of severe hypoglycaemia increases in children with impaired hypoglycaemia awareness. This may cause coma, seizures or death. These children are at high risk of severe hypoglycaemia with considerable morbidity and mortality.

Management

1. The use of real-time CGM with predictive alarms in addition to insulin pump therapy may be considered to reduce hypoglycaemia in such patients
2. Hypoglycaemia unawareness should be addressed with revision of hypoglycaemia prevention and management and frequent self-monitoring.
3. Hypoglycaemia awareness can be restored in some patients by periods of complete avoidance of hypoglycaemia, and by increasing the lower limit of their target.
4. In very young and very insulin-sensitive children, making insulin dose adjustments can be very difficult, especially if they have impaired hypoglycaemia awareness. Insulin pump therapy should be considered as it will allow smaller insulin dosage delivery and basal rates to be finely controlled to requirements

Glycaemic variability

When referring to human pathology the term variability is often used in a negative sense. However, variability plays a fundamental role in all of the primary control systems in our body. The circadian rhythm of the hormones involved in glucose metabolism has been related to variations in blood glucose levels. Glycaemic variability is not always negative because changes in blood glucose levels are the physiological consequence of hormones involved in the control of glucose metabolism and carbohydrate intake.

Increased swings in the severity of blood glucose are called glucose variability. High frequency of glucose variations was shown to increasethe risk of diabetes related vascular complications.

Remember that glucose variability is not reflected by the HbA1c, as the average glucose may not be high, and can be missed in intermittent blood glucose testing. Mismatch between insulin and carbohydrates may cause significant variability and this can be reduced by structured education to support carbohydrate counting.CGM may identify increased glycaemic variability and, in conjunction with insulin, food and detailed activity diaries may help to find the reasons behind it. The standard deviation of glucose is often reported from CGM traces and is the simplest method of assessing variability; a normal value is around 1.5 mmol/L (27 mg/dl).

Dawn effect

An insulin pump can be effective in managing the dawn effect without causing hypoglycaemia. It increases insulin to be delivered during the early hours of the morning. Higher basal rates (20–30%) from around 02:00am are advised.

We may need to increase ICR at breakfast. With a pump, such calculations can be accommodated using the bolus calculator.

Frequent overnight testing can be very inconvenient for children with diabetes. CGM provides a convenient way to assess and improve overnight glycaemic control and often reveals issues not noted previously. You may also need to consider revising management of hypoglycaemia with your patient/parents.

Dusk phenomenon

Remember, no interventions to address these phenomena will produce more problems. To manage Dusk phenomenon we need to regulate up insulin dosage before dinner by insulin pump to control hyperglycaemia.

3.10 Coming off the pump

Remember that a child without diabetes never goes without insulin. Many children or parents of children on a pump ask if they should disconnect their pump during exercise, swimming and in other situations. This depends on individual comfort and the specific situation. We should work with patients to develop an appropriate plan of action to minimise the impact on BG control for their particular sport or situation.

Indications:

1- Pump failure
2- Changing to subcutaneous injections
3- Patient dislikes the pump (rare)
4- Occasionally for specific sports (swimming, boxing and rugby)
5- Pump holiday
6- Parties: wedding and other occasions where patient doesn't like others to see a device attached to their bodies.

To work out how much long-acting basal insulin is needed – the following approximation may be used:
1- Calculate total daily basal insulin on the pump programme.
2- Increase this by 20% to determine the amount of long-acting insulin needed per day (a 30% increase may be needed, but a conservative 20% increase is advised at first).
3- This can be given as one or two doses, depending on which insulin is being used and total insulin dose.
4- The pump should be discontinued 2 h after the first long-acting insulin injection is given. It is best to do this in the morning to minimise the risk of problems at night.
5- Bolus insulin and corrective doses should be taken as usual. If a bolus calculator is used, the one on the pump can still be used or a calculator integrated into a capillary blood glucose meter can be used.

Resuming pump therapy

When resuming pump treatment, return to previous pump settings. The best time to restart is just before the long-acting insulin has worn off (approximately 2 h prior to the next due dose of long-acting insulin). It is advisable not to do this just before bedtime as close monitoring is advisable after re-starting pump treatment.

4 Insulin pump and food

    4.1   Carbohydrate and glycaemic index
    4.2   Advanced bolus options

4.1 Carbohydrate and glycaemic index

Because carbohydrates have the biggest impact on blood glucose, insulin dose should be matched with food intake to get the best results from the pump. Carbohydrate counting provides an accurate and flexible approach that is particularly suited to fast-acting insulin analogues and pumps. This is particularly important if your patient uses the 'bolus calculator' on their pump.

Carbohydrate counting allows us to provide the pump with the right information. If you put the wrong information in, you will get the wrong calculation from the pump. CHO is counted in grams (g) for pump therapy. Even if they have been counting CHO for a while, it is worth having a refresher session with the child's dietician before starting with the pump to ensure everything is up to date. Food that needs to be counted are those containing starch CHO, those containing natural sugars and those containing added sugars, as shown in Table 4.1.

There are a few ways of counting CHO, including using food labels, weighing foods, measuring cups and spoons, using nutritional books, using phone apps and using recipes.

A. Weighing foods

Weighing foods is the most accurate way to count CHO in foods without labels, or when the portion size varies. The best example of the foods that are good to weigh includes rice, couscous, noodles, pasta, potatoes (chips, jacket, roast, mashed,), fruits and breakfast cereals.

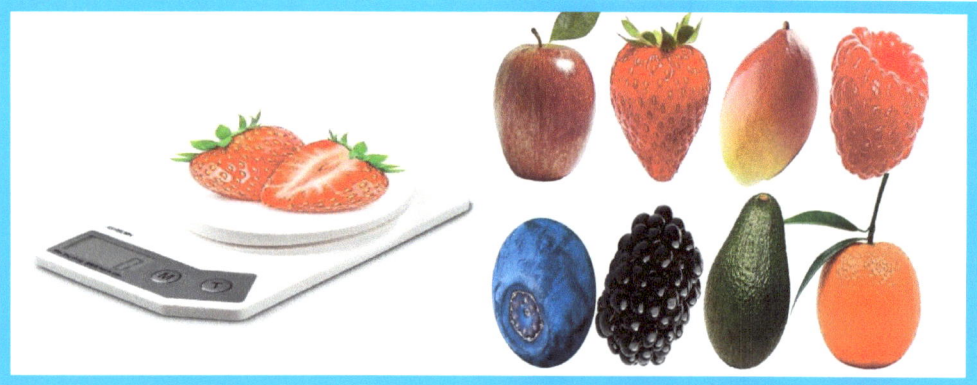

Figure 4.1

Pre-programmed scales that come with the nutritional values of foods can calculate the CHO value based on the weight of food. However, a pair of digital scales (Figure 4.1) and some maths will do the same job!

To calculate how much CHO in a portion of weighed food, find out how much CHO in 100g of food and divide by 100. Multiply the result by the weighed portion size (g).

Food weighing on digital scales will help your patient become familiar with what the serving size looks like and be more accurate when estimating their serve size.
Keep a record of the child's portion sizes of different foods to avoid having to reweigh each time. However, reweigh portions every three to six months to check the new CHO contents because children's portion sizes change as they grow.

B. Using food labels

The label on a food gives values per 100 grams and/or per portion. To calculate the net carbs in whole foods, subtract the fiber and protein from the total number of carbohydrates. The label on some food packaging only gives the sugar value, therefore you need to use the 'total carbohydrate' figure, NOT the 'of which sugars' figure.

If you are weighing food, you can use the 'per 100 g' figure. The 'per portion' value is useful for quantities you can easily count.

Table 4.1 Food that needs to be counted

Food containing starchy CHO	Food containing natural sugars
<ul><li>Bread</li><li>breakfast cereals</li><li>bread products and items containing flour</li><li>bulgar wheat</li><li>cassava</li><li>chapattis</li><li>couscous</li><li>crackers</li><li>noodles</li><li>potatoes</li><li>pasta</li><li>parsnips</li></ul>	<ul><li>dried fruit</li><li>drinking yoghurt</li><li>fruits</li><li>fruit juice</li><li>fruit smoothies</li><li>milk</li><li>milkshake</li><li>rice pudding</li><li>yoghurt</li></ul>
	Food containing added sugars

• pastry • pulse vegetables (baked beans, mushy peas, other beans, peas, chickpeas, dahl, lentils) • quinoa • rice • yams • squashes • sweet potato	• biscuits • brownies • cakes • cheesecake • chocolate • chocolate biscuits • cookies • doughnuts • ice cream • mousse • muffins • sweets • other desserts

Fats and plain proteins are not counted (although they may slow CHO absorption).
On some food labels, the grams of dietary fiber are already included in the total carbohydrate count, but because fiber is a type of carbohydrate that our body can't digest, the fiber does not increase blood sugar levels.

C. Using recipes

Recipes can be used to count carbohydrates in food. You need to work out the whole recipe then divide it by number of portions:

> Quantity (g) multiplied by grams of CHO/100 g then Gram CHO/100 g multiplied by quantity.

D. Books

There are many books available to help count calories. Some also contain CHO values. Some books give values some per portion (useful when the patients are out or away from home); per 100 g (useful for weighing) and some have photos to show different quantities. Below are some examples:
   1- Carbs & Cals by Chris Cheyette and Yello Balolia.
   2- Calorie Counter by Colins Gem.

E. Phone applications

Some CHO counting books are also available as apps.
Carbs & Cals book is also available as an app

F. Carbohydrate reference lists

These are an alternative when a nutrition label is not available. Lists are easily available online, from structured learning programmes, books or nutrition reference and Smartphone apps. In these programmes a variety of popular foods are usually included.

Example 1
A 12-year-old boy with a blood glucose level of 180 mg/dl, target 96 mg/dl, eating one medium banana (20 g CHO) and one small apple (15 g CHO). His ICR is 1 unit:10 g (ICR is 10) and his ISF is 1 unit:45 mg/dl (ISF is 45). Calculate how much insulin is required.

Answer:
Carbohydrate content of food = 20 g (banana) + 15 g (apple) = 35 g.
Insulin needed for food = total carbohydrate eaten ÷ ICR = 35 ÷ 10 = 3.5 units
Insulin needed for correction of high glucose = (current glucose−target glucose)/ISF = (180-96)/45 = 1.8 units
Total insulin = bolus for food + corrective dose = 3.5 + 1.8 =5.3 units

---

Example 2
A 16-year-old girl with a blood glucose level of 100 mg/dl, target 100 mg/dl, eating four pizza slices (120 g CHO). Her ICR is 1 unit:10 g and her ISF is 1 unit:45 mg/dl. How much insulin does she require?

Answer:
Carbohydrate content of food = 120 g
Insulin needed for food = total carbohydrates eaten × ICR = 120 ÷ 10 = 12 units
Insulin needed for correction of high glucose = (current glucose-target glucose)/ISF = zero
Total insulin = bolus for food + corrective dose = 12 units

This is a large meal with high fat food and delayed absorption expected, therefore we should use a dual/multi-wave bolus option like: 6 units now (normal bolus) and 6 units over 4 h (extended or square wave bolus).

We need to consider the following points when counting CHO:

1. Serving size: in certain foods, this can be done easily, for example with fruit, pizza slices or bread slices. In other foods it can be more difficult and requires objective accurate measurements with food measures. This is usually the case for foods like rice, pasta, cereals and mashed potato, which are difficult to quantify with the eye alone and are rich in carbohydrate content. Food scales, measuring cups and spoons can be used. The carbohydrate values of cooked and raw foods can vary.
2. Remember precise measurements mean more correct insulin doses and any measurement errors can affect blood glucose.
3. Correct ISF, ICR and basal: these should be calculated accurately.
4. Food label: Calculation of the carbohydrate in the serving size should be done, because carbohydrate amounts are often expressed as 100 g of food rather than serving size.
5. Good simple arithmetic skills and/or a calculator are required for carbohydrate counting, to work out carbohydrate content and insulin doses.
6. Practice is necessary to get the best results from CHO counting. It may not work the first few times but does get easier.
7. Refresher courses are essential to maintain CHO counting skills.
8. Frequent blood glucose monitoring and accurate record-keeping are essential, to understand whether the approach is working or needs adjusting. A few attempts may be needed to ensure it is working correctly.
9. Use the pump correctly: remember that even with rapid-acting insulin, the optimal time to bolus is around 10-15 min before food.
10. Always consider other variables that may strongly effect on insulin action, such as illness, activity and exercise, fasting, growth spurts and menstrual periods.
11. Test your patients' CHO ration every 6-8 weeks.
12. Plan for your road trips.
13. Learn from mistakes and ask for help when needed.
14. Regular follow up with Dietician and other healthcare professionals for further support.

Glycaemic Index (GI)

GI is a relative ranking of carbohydrate in foods according to how they affect blood glucose levels. The lower the GI, the slower the rise in blood glucose levels will be when the food is consumed. Carbohydrates with a low GI value (55 or less) are slowly digested, absorbed and metabolised and cause a lower and slower rise in blood glucose.

Each CHO food is given a value. It is scored on a scale of 100, with pure glucose being 100. Slowly-absorbed foods have a low GI rating, typically <55. Food quickly absorbed have a high GI rating, typically >75. High-value GI foods are broken down very quickly, causing a rapid increase in blood glucose levels.

There are many lists for glycaemic index. GI is affected by many factors (including cooking, processing, physical form, acidity, fat or fibre content). GI can also be affected by individual variation in speed of digestion with high pre-meal glucose and large meals also slowing digestion. Therefore, learning lists are not of great value, however, it is useful to recognize the GI index as a variable when assessing post-meal glucose values, choosing type and amount of bolus and when adjusting insulin times.

Dietary fats, fibre and protein

Fat and protein, in foods or as part of a meal may slow the release of sugar from CHO foods and reduce the GI. Dietary fats may contribute to delayed increases in glucose levels by slowing the absorption of food. We recommend that once you have achieved good control with your patient's basal rate and bolusing with meals, you may want to fine-tune that control by looking at meals specifically high in fats (e.g. fish and chips, pizza, creamy curries and pasta dishes). In very compliant patients this might be the only cause of their high blood glucose.

You may find that their blood glucose stays higher than you would have predicted for a longer period of time after these types of meals. If so, discuss with the dietitian and consider a different bolus type or a temporary basal rate increase for up to 8 hours. Pizza or curry are an example of high fat meals, especially if consumed in large quantities. They can slow digestion, resulting in longer absorption times for carbohydrates.

A high-fat meal can also result in the body being more resistant to insulin after several hours. Therefore, after a high-fat meal, glucose tends to rise later. That's why a normal immediate bolus could result in an initial fall in glucose, followed by delayed hyperglycaemia. The dual- or multi-wave bolus option is one of the ways to overcome this problem, usually taking anywhere between 30% and 70% of the bolus amount immediately and the remaining over 2–4 hours.

Fibre is not digested and therefore not turned to glucose. If >5 g of a serving is coming from fibre, subtract fibre from the total carbohydrate content.

Amino acids which make up protein can be metabolized to form new glucose molecules, particularly during periods of fasting. This can result in glucose rises several hours after a meal. Protein may also have a protective effect, reducing the frequency of post-meal hypoglycaemia. Carbohydrate-free protein snacks and meals may need a small insulin bolus but there is no validated way to calculate the insulin to protein ratio.

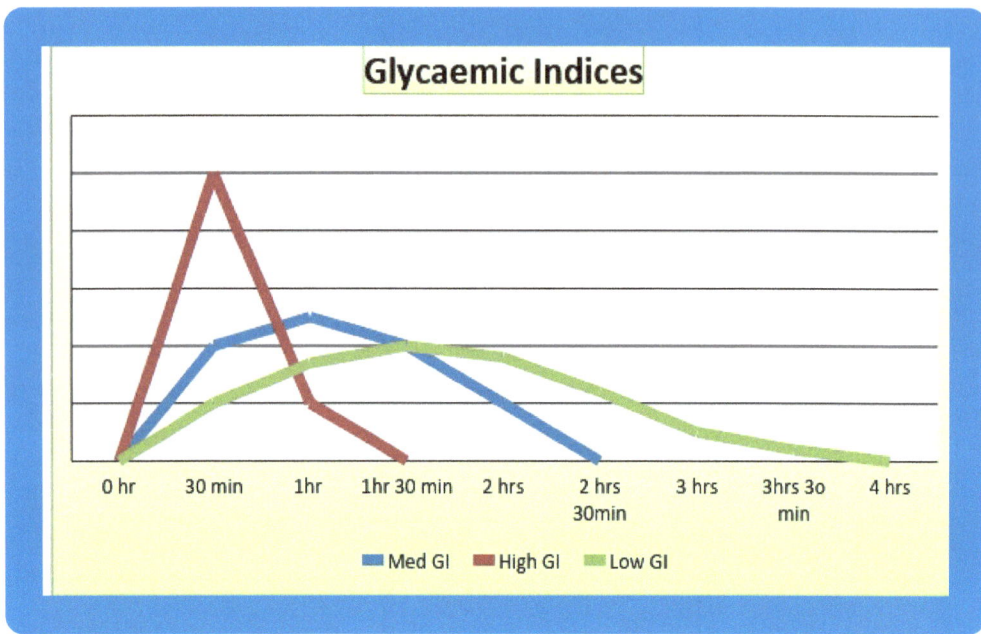

Figure 4.2 Glycaemic indicies

Tackling problems caused by differences in glycaemic indices of the food:

1- Including more naturally low GI foods in the child's diet will help smooth out his/her blood glucose readings and maintain energy levels between meals.
2- Different bolus patterns should be used with mixed meals to slow the insulin delivery to match the release of sugar from CHO foods.
3- Most main meals (which contain protein and fat) benefit from using a dual or combination wave bolus over one to four hours.
4- A dual wave bolus could also be beneficial for some meals containing both quick and slow release CHO. This delivers some insulin quickly and some insulin over one to four hours. The percentage of quickly and slowly delivered insulin depends on what you set, but usual combinations are 70:30, 50:50 or 30:70.

5- Patients eating a meal that contains fat, protein and low GI CHO may need to extend their bolus over four to six hours, e.g. 50:50 or 30:70. Trial, error and good record keeping is required to get this right.
6- To get the best match you also need to discuss this with your dietitian.

4.2 Advanced bolus options

Insulin pumps have the ability to deliver different bolus types. The names may differ from one pump to another, however there are three main types of boluses:
a- standard or normal
b- square or extended wave
c- dual wave, multi-wave or combination.

a- Standard or normal

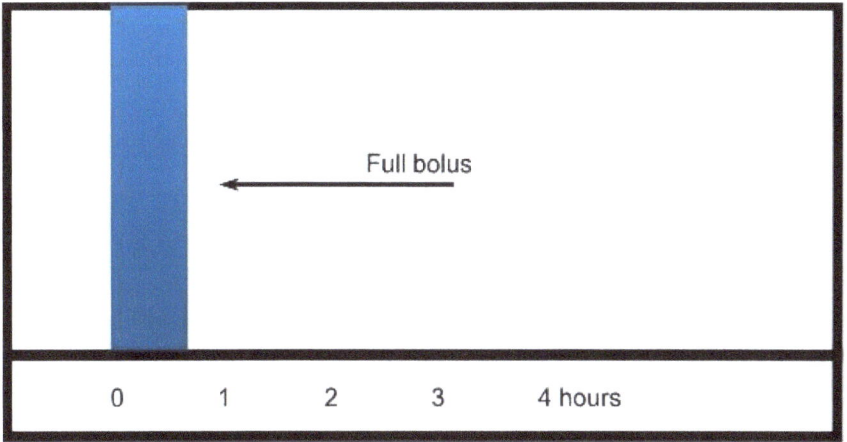

Figure 4.3 Standard bolus

In standard type, the whole bolus is given straight away. Sometimes we do not know how much food the child is going to eat, in this situation we could give two normal boluses close together; some before they eat and then a top up when they have finished eating and we know how much more to give.

b- Square or extended wave

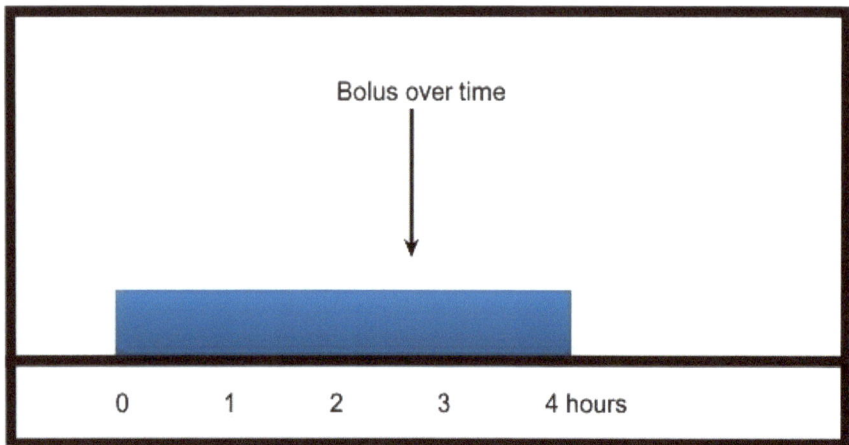

Figure 4.4 Extended bolus

In an extended or square wave bolus the total bolus is spread out over time. The whole dose is evenly spread over the choice of time (15 minutes to eight hours). It is useful for long spread-out meals, buffets and meals with either a very high fat or low glycaemic index content. It can be stopped at any time.

This option can be programmed to match the rise in blood glucose following a high fat meal that takes longer to be absorbed, e.g. fish and chips, pasta with cheese sauce, curries (especially with bread and rice), pizza (especially with meat or extra cheese topping).

c- Multiwave, dual wave or combination

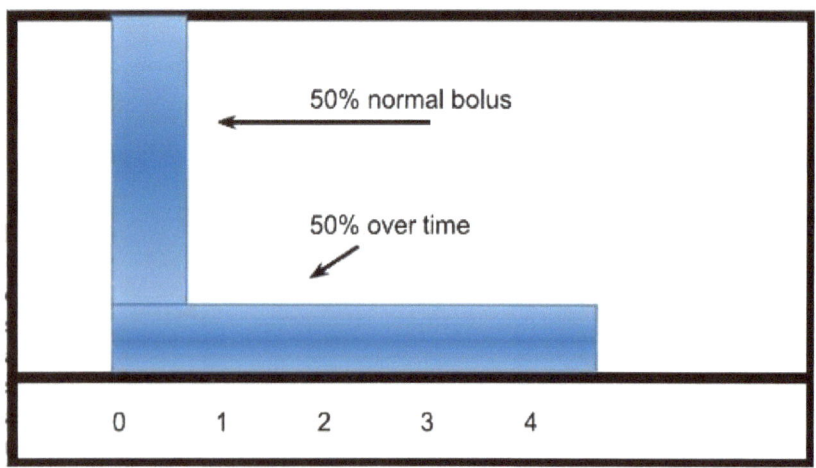

Figure 4.5 Combined bolus

A combination of the normal and extended wave is called multi or dual wave. In this case, a chosen amount is given immediately and the rest over time. This is useful for most meals containing fats, protein and CHO.

A dual wave bolus can be given as half immediately and half over a period of time (50:50), or in any other ratio (30:70, 70:30).

Bolus calculators

Insulin bolus calculation is needed several times per day and is challenging and resource-demanding. Bolus insulin equations are complex and—for some patients—difficult and time consuming to solve. Therefore, bolus calculators are essential to support patients in insulin treatment decisions. Bolus calculators are available integrated in all insulin pumps, in the form of software applications that can be downloaded to Smartphones and as separate devices. Bolus calculators are an effective way of ensuring consistency as your patient gradually takes on more responsibility.

Your patient's personal settings, such as: blood glucose target, insulin sensitivity factor (ISF), insulin to CHO ratio (ICR), insulin on board (IOB) or 'active insulin' can be programmed into the pump. You can have different settings for different times of the day.

Bolus calculators account for insulin on board and reduce the risk of hypoglycaemia. A dose will be suggested but remember that your patient will still need to complete a pre-meal blood glucose test and calculate and enter the amount of CHO. You also still need to consider type and amount of CHO, environmental temperature, exercise and individual variability in absorption for different age groups.

These settings need to be reviewed every two to three months, or whenever there is a need, such as when the family starts to feel less confident in the advice given by the bolus calculator.

Bolus use and frequent snacks

A 'saw tooth' appearance on CGM can be caused by frequent snacks that contain carbohydrate. This can be challenging to manage. Frequent rapid-acting insulin bolus doses increase the risk of hypoglycaemia due to insulin stacking. Insufficient insulin with snacks may lead to hyperglycaemia. Bolus advice calculators, especially those integrated into insulin pumps, will include insulin on-board in their calculations and help to optimise glucose with snacks.

To resolve the problem of frequent snacks and bolus use try the following:
1- Look at the pump download (to review frequency of boluses and timing in relation to food).
2- Revise carbohydrate counting, review insulin:carbohydrate ratios and support boluses at the time of snacks.
3- Try basal rate testing and adjustment without influence of snacks.
4- Consider carbohydrate-free snack options and reduce frequency of snacking.

Insulin on Board (IOB)

Pumps have a feature that allows us to track the rate at which your body uses your bolus insulin (insulin on board). Even with rapid-acting insulin, your body takes some time to use your entire bolus insulin. IOB is designed to safely give a correction bolus between meals without stacking your insulin.

When the IOB feature is activated, your pump tracks and displays how much of that bolus is still working to lower your BG. You can activate IOB and set your personal IOB duration in the Advanced Setup menu. The pump will track each bolus over the period of time that you programmed it for. It will use this data to calculate and recommend a reduced bolus dose.

Points to remember:
- The duration setting for IOB is the point at which insulin is finished working in your body.
- You can customize the time frame so that IOB will track your bolus doses, ranging from 2.0 hours to 6.0 hours.
- IOB only tracks bolus insulin. Basal insulin is NOT involved in IOB tracking or calculations.
- IOB will track all bolus doses you take for a given amount of time.
- This setting varies from person to person and can be affected by other factors.
- Patient should be advised on an appropriate time frame suitable for him/her.
- If BG is below target, IOB is subtracted from carbohydrate boluses (if you are entering carbohydrate and a low BG).
- When BG is above target, IOB will only be subtracted from BG (or correction) boluses, NOT from carbohydrate boluses.
- If you change the battery, any IOB will be cleared. The pump cannot detect how long a battery is out, so it cannot accurately track how much insulin is still on board.

In summary, the pump is great at calculating your patients' bolus doses, but they still need to think for themselves. For example, IOB doesn't know what type of meal you had last. What if it was high-fat meal? Sometimes, even with a significant amount of IOB and a BG in your target range, you may still see a higher BG later if you ate high-fat foods and/or foods with slower-digesting carbohydrate. The pump also doesn't know their activity level.

5 Life with an insulin pump

- 5.1 School and social Life
- 5.2 Activity and exercise
- 5.3 Illness
- 5.4 Hospital admission for surgeries and severe illness.
- 5.5 Holidays and travel
- 5.6 Ramadan and fasting
- 5.7 Stressful and unplanned situations
- 5.8 Puberty and menstruation
- 5.9 Coffee and alcohol
- 5.10 Steroids
- 5.11 Psychological aspects of insulin pump therapy

5.1 School and social life

School

Parents should inform the school of their child's diagnosis as soon as possible, to enable them to prepare for their child returning to school. Management of diabetes in school requires communication between healthcare professionals, school staff and carers, to ensure effective and safe diabetes control during school time. Insulin pump therapy can be self-managed by many children at a young age but, in case of pump failure, insulin should be kept at school in a fridge with needles and syringe or insulin pen, and school staff should be familiar with hyper and hypoglycaemia treatment.

Moving from MDI to insulin pump is usually planned in advance, therefore, it is a good idea to show the staff at the child's school the pump ahead of time.

The child's diabetes nurse will explain what it is, how it works and the key differences compared to an MDI regime, particularly when more immediate action is required. The school nurse needs to be informed about the recommended list of supplies that should be kept at school. Parents/carers may need to take few days off work in case they get called by the school nurse. The school nurse will probably not be involved in placing and replacing infusion sets, but it is important for them to know the basic information about the infusion set and to recognise if an infusion set is not working properly.

Social life

Ask any child, and you'll likely hear that time spent with friends is the most important part of the school day. It is important that a child using a pump is able to make friends and participate in parties. He or she should be able to enjoy the same games and eat the same reasonably-healthy party food as everyone else.

Family members, close friends and school nurses should be engaged in understanding how to manage a child's diabetes and insulin pump.

Many children enjoy parties and sleeping over at a friend's house. It is important that the friend's parent feels confident with blood glucose monitoring, pump basics, recognition of tube kinking, pump failure and management of hyper- and hypoglycaemia. It is a good idea to write them a list of instructions

If the child is going to be involved in a new situation such as travelling abroad, a festival, sleepover, etc., it is important to discuss how they will handle it in advance. Discuss with your patients/parents the additional options available, like setting a temporary basal for managing these types of situation while on insulin pump therapy.

Sleeping, swimming and showering

The pump can be placed in a pocket, clipped to pyjamas or under the pillow.

Pump users can shower and swim with the pump. Most pumps are waterproof. However, ensure your battery cap is not cracked or broken.

Although it is okay to swim or shower with the pump, extreme temperatures (very hot water) can affect the quality of insulin. So, it is advised not to wear it in a hot tub or hot bath.

5.2 Activity and exercise

We often need less insulin during and after activity, and therefore the option to decrease the basal rate is useful.

During exercise, the glucose consumption increases to meet the increased energy demands from the muscles. Intense exercise can lead to a very dramatic consumption of glucose, especially in the first 15 minutes. There is also an increase in the skin blood flow, which accelerates insulin absorption and increases the risk of hypoglycaemia during exercise.

Each child reacts differently to activity, therefore adjusting insulin rates for activity is often a process of trial and error.

Exercise increases the sensitivity of muscle to insulin, making it more responsive to insulin and glucose consumption is higher as it replenishes its glycogen stores. Therefore, there is an increased risk of hypoglycaemia following exercise and insulin requirements are reduced for up to 24 hours.

The extent of exercise effect on glycaemic control depends on the duration and intensity of exercise. Anaerobic or very intense exercise can cause a paradoxical rise in blood glucose mediated by adrenaline and counter-regulatory hormones to insulin during and after exercise.

Hyperglycaemia during exercise adversely affects muscle performance and there is an increased risk of dehydration and ketosis. Aerobic exercise usually results in a reduction in blood glucose, whereas anaerobic exercise increases adrenaline levels and may cause a rise in blood glucose.

Activity and exercise are essential for children with diabetes. However, insulin delivery adjustments are required before, during and after activity to avoid hypo- and hyperglycaemic excursions; this is easier when managed with pumps.

Activities combining both forms of exercise, coupled with competition stress and excitement can have variable effects. Remember that the risk of hypoglycaemia following aerobic exercise may persist for many hours and even into the next day; therefore, insulin dose adjustment may need to continue overnight until the next morning. Remember that one episode of hypoglycaemia increases the risk of subsequent hypoglycaemia, which may be further exacerbated by exercise. It is advised to avoid exercise for 12 -24 hours after a hypoglycaemic episode.

Hypoglycaemia during exercise may lead to loss of confidence and prevents participation in further activities. Reduced confidence regarding exercise is a frequent problem in children with diabetes. Activity should be encouraged and CGM can be a very useful adjunct for children with diabetes who exercise frequently. CGM can help achieve better control, performance and confidence.

Points to consider when exercising:
1- Check BG before (2 h prior and immediately before), during (30–60 min into exercise) and after activity to establish your specific patterns. Keep written records.
2- If BG is 14.0 mmol/L (250 mg/dl) or greater prior to exercise, check for ketones. Treat this problem. Advise your patients to avoid exercise if they have ketones.
3- Start slowly and build up. As tolerance improves, and the body's strength and glycogen stores increase, you may find that the body responds differently.
4- Avoid exercise if you have had hypoglycaemia in the last 12 hrs.
5- Advise your patients to keep their 'Hypo Kit' with them at all times.
6- Drink plenty of water to stay well hydrated.
7- Plan ahead: it is a good idea to set a temporary basal, reduce insulin bolus and take some carbohydrate before predictable exercise.
8- Remember, competitive short duration exercise may not need an immediate reduction in insulin and may even require a corrective bolus after exercise. However, after exercise there is a risk of delayed hypoglycaemia, this can be minimised with carbohydrate ingestion and insulin reduction.

9- Reduction of basal insulin following exercise (in this case a temporary basal rate of 60–80%) would be advised.
10- Patients should wear medical identification.
11- Try the same exercise at different times of the day to see if glucose response differs.
12- In general, exercise lasting longer than 30 minutes will require extra carbohydrate or a decrease in insulin.
13- Adjust the insulin that has the greatest effect during the exercise session: basal insulin or the bolus dose.
14- When adjusting your basal insulin, begin 60-90 minutes before the activity, if you can.
15- If exercising within an hour or two of a bolus, decrease the bolus. However, if your exercise is not close to a bolus, consider a basal adjustment using the Temporary Basal Rate.
16- You may find adjusting both basal and bolus insulin is best when exercising for long durations.
17- Remember, because of the "lag effect" of exercise, you may need to decrease insulin for as long as 24-36 hours after the exercise. This is especially true for activities that last for several hours.

Approaches to prevent hypoglycaemia during exercise

1 – Reduce temporary basal rate
Basal insulin levels can be reduced prior to, during and after a period of exercise.
Reduce basal insulin by up to 50%, start 60–120 min before exercise and maintain the reduction during the exercise.

Exercise intensity and examples	Light activity: short bike riding, walking	Moderate activity: football, swimming, dance class, cricket, rugby, jumping on a trampoline	Heavy activity: Boxing sessions, school residential trips, sport tournaments, weekend hiking
Bolus	No reduction	40- 50% reduction	50% reduction
Basal during exercise	10-30% reduction	40-50% reduction	50% reduction & eat CHO
Basal after exercise	No reduction	No reduction	30-50% reduction for up to 12 hours, occasionally longer

> All-day activity may require a 50% reduction in the basal rate during the day and 25% that night.

2 – Carbohydrate loading

Altering basal rates before exercise may not always be possible. Fast-acting carbohydrate immediately prior to intense, short activity may be helpful. For longer, moderate intensity, a slow-releasing solid snack may be better. Take 15–20 g extra carbohydrates without an insulin bolus before exercise.

3 – Reduced bolus

Take a reduced bolus with meals prior to exercise. If eating a meal within 2 hours prior to exercise, reduce the bolus dose by 25–75%. The above approaches may be used in combination. Personal preference, timing of exercise and blood glucose levels before exercise will dictate which one to use.

After exercise

The increased risk of hypoglycaemia after exercise can last for 24 hours. This may be problematic, especially overnight. Therefore, following any significant exercise, the following can be tried to prevent hypoglycaemia:

1. Check capillary blood glucose regularly after exercise.
2. Reduce temporary basal rate by 20–50% for 2–4 h.
3. For the next 24 h, a separate basal insulin setting with a smaller reduction (of around 20%) in basal insulin is advised. The biggest period of reduction is in the overnight basal rate.
4. The ICR following exercise may be reduced to reduce insulin boluses. Either 15–20 g extra carbohydrate or a 20% reduction in bolus insulin may be needed with the main meal following exercise.

Every child responds differently, therefore it is important to advise your patients to practice good record-keeping and have regular reviews to determine how the body responds to different types of activities.

Common issues during and after exercise:

A- Hyperglycaemia prior to activity

Hyperglycaemia prior to exercise can be due to stress, excitement or low insulin levels. The low insulin level will trigger the liver to release stored glucose. Since the insulin level is low, the extra glucose has no way to enter the cells and eventually ketones will be released as the body resorts to breaking down fat to meet the muscles' need for energy.

B- Immediate hypoglycaemia during or just after exercise

This is due to increased glucose consumption during exercise. Remember that exercise can mask the symptoms of hypoglycaemia such as sweating.

This problem can be solved by:
1- Reducing basal settings prior to exercise and ensure reduction is at least 60-90 min before exercise.
2- Take extra carbohydrate before or during exercise, depending on when the hypoglycaemia occurs.
3- Use continuous glucose sensing or test during the exercise period to get a better understanding of glucose change.

C- Delayed overnight hypoglycaemia

This can happen due to recovery and replenishment of glycogen with increased insulin sensitivity. It can be prevented by:
1- Further reduction of overnight basal.
2- Consider setting an alarm and testing during the night or using continuous monitoring.
3- If the hypoglycaemia is in the first half of the night, consider reducing dinner bolus or taking bedtime snacks.

D- Post-exercise hyperglycaemia

Anaerobic and intense activity may trigger stress responses. This could lead to hyperglycaemia after exercise. In some children, this may be very marked and can lead to dehydration, ketosis and can impair the recovery period after exercise.

To prevent this problem:
1- Keep well-hydrated during exercise.
2- Test immediately after exercise and take a correction insulin bolus, which may be higher than usual due to the presence of counter-regulatory hormones to insulin.
3- Minimise basal reductions during exercise, test during exercise and give a 50% corrective bolus if high to prevent high BG.

E- Issues with contact sports

The cannula or pump may be dislodged during some contact sports like boxing, kickboxing and rugby. Occasionally the pump can be broken.
Solution:
1- It is advised to remove the pump for periods up to an hour.

2- After an hour, test capillary blood glucose.
3- Take required carbohydrate and insulin and continue exercise.

F- Issues with swimming

Most new pumps can be worn when swimming and will deliver a basal throughout the activity.

To avoid any problems during swimming:
1- Removed pumps and cannulas can be left attached.
2- Remove the pump if swimming in a non-chlorinated environment to avoid risk of infection.
3- The cap for the cannula and a dressing can be worn if the child decides to leave the pump attached to the body.
4- If the pump is removed for over an hour, test capillary blood glucose, take required carbohydrate and insulin and continue swimming.

Questions to ask during clinic visit:

1- Do they need to take their pump off to participate in the activity?
2- Will they need an extra activity snack, or can it be managed by reducing their insulin dose with the meal bolus beforehand?
3- If they are wearing their pump, do they need to reduce their basal rate during the activity?
4- Will their basal rate need to be reduced after the activity and how long for?

5.3 Illness

Infections associated with a temperature often increase counter-regulatory stress hormone secretion. This will increase insulin requirements with an associated risk of hyperglycaemia (which can cause dehydration) and ketosis. However, there is a risk of hypoglycaemia in any illness with vomiting, diarrhoea or where there is poor oral intake.

In these circumstances, if bolus correction has failed and your patients' glucose levels remain above 14 mmol/l (250 mg/dl) consider increasing the basal rate over 4 to 12 hours (sometimes longer) to 120%. In some circumstances it may be necessary to gradually increase in steps up to 200%. You may find it useful to set a second basal pattern with an increase of 20% for the period of the illness.

The following general tips are helpful to pump users:

1. Never stop or suspend the pump.

2. You may need extra insulin for moderate or severe illnesses.
3. Try to eat simple, digestible foods if unable to tolerate complex meals. If you cannot eat, stay well-hydrated (little and often fluid intake).
4. Check blood glucose every 1–3 hours (more frequently in severe illnesses).
5. Check blood or urine ketones if blood sugar is above 14 mmol/L (250 mg/dl) or if you are vomiting, and treat when appropriate.
6. Keep a log of glucose, ketones, insulin, fluids and vomiting.
7. They should have pens or syringes to use in case pump failure.
8. Seek medical attention if vomiting persists, if continuing to have high ketones or glucose or if unable to eat and drink.
9. Patients need to let others know that they are unwell.
10. Be aware that some medications may also impact on glucose (e.g. steroids, which are used in acute exacerbations of eczema or asthma).

5.4 Hospital admission for surgeries and severe illnesses

When children with diabetes require sedation or anaesthesia for surgery or medical procedures, optimal management should maintain adequate hydration and near-to-normal glucose levels, while minimising the risk of hypoglycaemia. The stress of surgery may cause acute hyperglycaemia, which increases the risk of postoperative infection.

Where possible, children with type 1 diabetes on pump therapy should be empowered to continue self-management of their diabetes during hospital admissions. Healthcare professionals should be aware and comfortable with this.

Proper care and management should include:

- Diabetes management throughout surgery and post-operatively
- Avoidance of hypoglycaemia
- Avoidance of ketoacidosis (DKA)
- Minimising the duration of inpatient stay

A clear written procedure and guidelines should be provided for medical and nursing staff to follow when giving surgical care and management to children and young people with diabetes during their hospital stay.

Maintaining good glycaemic control in the preoperative period will reduce the risk of DKA/dehydration, hypoglycaemia and post-operative infections.

What to do about child's pump during hospital admission

1- If the child is having a major operation they will need to remove their pump and be given insulin intravenously.
2- If your patient is having a minor operation it may be possible for him/her to keep their pump on with the agreement of the anaesthetist.
3- If it is a planned admission, ensure you discuss it with your patients and/or parents beforehand.
4- We may need to adjust child's basal rate before admission. Often a 10-20% reduction from time of starvation is advised.
5- If the patient is admitted with high blood glucose levels or ketones, he/she should be asked to remove their pump and be given intravenous insulin until the problem has been resolved.
6- If the child is capable of looking after their diabetes themselves, they should continue using their pump while in hospital, provided they have the agreement of the medical team caring for them.
7- If the child is not able to look after their insulin pump themselves, you should use other methods to give insulin. Ensure your patient's pump is stored safely if taken off.
8- If pump therapy is discontinued or the pump is removed, subcutaneous basal insulin or intravenous insulin infusion must be used.
9- DKA should be managed according to local guidelines. It is important to ensure that pump failure or problems with insulin delivery via the pump are not the cause of DKA. If the insulin pump was disconnected, the pump can be restarted once the DKA has been treated (avoid starting this overnight). Intravenous insulin infusion should be continued for a further 1–2 hours before stopping.

Procedures

1- Outpatient procedures: no adjustments may be needed if basal rates are set up correctly. Blood glucose should be monitored closely, as insulin requirements may go up (due to stress of the procedure) and sometimes fall (due to missed meals and if basal rates were not correct).

2- Elective surgery: basal insulin via pump may be continued but careful consideration of management of the pump while under anaesthetic is required. A variable rate intravenous insulin infusion should be considered. Factors in the operating theatre, such as diathermy and its impact on the pump, may influence this decision. For emergency surgery, it is likely to be safest to stop insulin pump therapy, store the pump safely and commence a variable rate intravenous insulin infusion.

General advice for all preoperative surgery

- Wherever possible, all patients should have a planned date for surgery.
- As a general rule, in all cases the child with diabetes must be first on the list in the morning.
- Ward staff to liaise with anaesthetist/surgeon and diabetes team following pre-admission assessment of diabetic patient.
- Parents should be advised to bring all of their child's insulin and blood testing meters with them to hospital.
- Patients should be encouraged to self-monitor their blood glucose levels and to self-inject their insulin.
- Careful and regular monitoring of blood glucose is required throughout the pre- and post-operative period.
- The aim is to optimise glycaemic control of between 5-10 mmol (90-180 mg/dl) during the stay in hospital.

Post-operative care – morning list

Inform parents that the child's blood glucose levels may run slightly higher than normal through the rest of the day and they may need to liaise with the diabetes team prior to or after discharge home.

Emergency surgery

An acute illness can commonly precipitate diabetic ketoacidosis, which may be present as an acute abdomen. The measurement of blood glucose and ketones is essential in all children with diabetes who are unwell for whatever reason.

Diabetes management must not be overlooked if child is a victim of trauma.

5.5 Holidays and travel

Travelling with a pump is slightly different and requires planning. Patients can go through security wearing their pump but should not let their pump go through the baggage X-ray machines.

Checklist for travelling:

1. For travel in hot countries or long-distance travel, keep insulin in an insulation bag, such as an evaporative cooling case.
2. Ensure you have all supplies – pump supplies and insulin, blood glucose and ketone monitors, fast- and long-acting insulin pens or syringe and glucagon kit.
3. Keep supplies in a bag that stays with the child at all times (cabin baggage). Batteries, infusion sets and extra pump reservoirs can be kept in check-in luggage.
4. Insulin should not be packed in a suitcase, as it is too cold in the hold and the luggage containing the medication could be lost.
5. Give a smaller back-up supply to someone travelling with the child in case luggage is misplaced
6. Keep a medical report stating that patient has type 1 diabetes, is on a pump, needs to carry supplies with him/her and needs to wear the pump at all times – . this may be needed for airport security.
7. Obtaining pump supplies can be difficult in some countries, know where to obtain medical help if needed and keep helpline and emergency contact numbers.
8. Keep a reminder record for important information the patient may need, such as pump settings, multiple dose injection doses and sick-day rules.
9. If travelling in a group, ensure group members are aware that the child has diabetes and what they may need to do in an emergency.

Basal insulin adjustments when travelling

One problem insulin-treated children with diabetes face when flying across time zones is confusion about how to adjust their insulin times and dosage amounts. The pump (and blood glucose meter) clocks should be adjusted to change the basal rates but it may take several days for circadian rhythms to adjust to a new time zone. Therefore, variable basal rates to match circadian patterns may initially be timed incorrectly.

Time zones

Be aware of the changes that should be made if your patient is flying to a different time zone.

1. If the new time zone is less than four hours different, adjust your patient's pump clock on arrival.
2. If the time zone is more than four hours different you can either:
    a- Use the lowest flat basal rate during flights, use correction doses if necessary and change time on arrival or departure according to

preference. Frequent capillary blood glucose testing will be required initially. Give boluses with meals as usual. Monitor blood glucose levels regularly and correct high and low readings as needed.

b- Adjust your patient's pump clock by three to four hours on departure and then gradually adjust further over the next few days.

You may need extra attention in the following situations:
    a. There is significant baseline variability in basal rates – such as for marked dawn phenomenon.
    b. There is reduced hypoglycaemia awareness or a history of recurrent or severe hypoglycaemia.

3. One strategy to optimize adjustment to a new time zone is to make pump clock adjustments in stages – by 2-3 h/day – and use a lower basal setting with frequent self-monitoring.

5.6 Ramadan and fasting

Fasting may be necessary when testing basal rate with insulin pump therapy, before surgical procedures, or may be a personal choice. The challenge for the patient and the physician is to manage diabetes without an interruption to fasting by avoiding hypoglycaemia and simultaneously ensuring that blood glucose remain at acceptable safe levels. Reductions in basal insulin, careful monitoring and avoiding bolus insulin may be required to maintain safe glucose levels. CGM can be a useful adjunct to support fasting.

Ramadan

During Ramadan, Muslims fast (no food or drink) from dawn to sunset each day for a month (29-30 days). The main risks of fasting for patients with diabetes include hypoglycaemia, hyperglycaemia, diabetic ketoacidosis and dehydration. This can be due to the change in timings of food, sleep and medications. Fasting during Ramadan with the help of sensor-augmented pump therapy avoids hypoglycaemia. CGM can be a very useful adjunct during fasting to maintain optimal glucose control and include reduction in basal insulin during the day.

Suggested guidelines for children fasting in Ramadan:

1. Keep hydrated by drinking water from the time you break your fast until Suhoor to prevent dehydration.
2. Apply a 40-50% reduction in basal profile between dawn and sunset.

3. Reduce basal 2-3 hours before sunset to avoid hypoglycaemia.
4. Increase ICR at end of fast meal (same as for breakfast). Counter-regulatory hormones may be high at the time the fast is broken and may require increased insulin.
5. Stable control is important to minimise the increased hypoglycaemia risk.
6. Hyperglycaemia is particularly hazardous, as during fasting people cannot drink and can become dehydrated.
7. The fast must be broken if there is:
    - Hypoglycemia: Blood glucose is 4mmol/l (70 mg/dl) or below and/or show symptoms of hypoglycaemia.
    - Hyperglycaemia: Blood glucose level higher than 16mmol/l (300 mg/dl), as they are at risk of dehydration.
    - They are nauseous and vomiting, or have any other severe illness.
8. Set a low alert: A higher value for the low glucose threshold (4.5 mmol/L in this case) during fasting is sensible, as it gives time for a temporary basal reduction to take effect (at least 60 min), since the intake of glucose to improve glucose levels is not possible during a fast.
9. A lower alarm rate at night prevents the sensor from alarming too frequently (which can result in alarm fatigue).
10. Eat low-GI foods and small portions.
11. Space out and balance meals.
12. Monitor blood glucose.

5.7 Stressful and unplanned situations

Stress, whether physical or mental, has been proven to induce changes in diabetes control, both directly and indirectly, which can be problematic.
Mental stress can causes the body to produce especially high levels of stress hormones, which drive blood sugar levels up. Patients are under stress, may skip meals or forget to take their medication, which will affect their blood sugar level.

Stressful situations are counter-regulatory to insulin action. Being told you have diabetes can also cause a lot of stress and pressure. This can make it harder to control blood sugar levels, which in most cases only adds to the frustration and stress.

Stress in children can be due to travel or to hospital admissions for minor or major operations. Family issues like sickness, separation, divorce and death in the family are major stress factors for children. There is significant interpersonal variation in how blood glucose reacts to the same stress, in direction, magnitude and duration of glucose change.

Management during stress:

1- Short-duration stress can be managed by a temporary basal increase 1-2 h before the event, if it can be anticipated. Increases may be conservative in children (10–20%) to avoid hypoglycaemia, which can impair performance. Additional small correction boluses can be used to address any remaining hyperglycaemia.

2- Long-duration stress may should be managed by:
A- Setting a higher basal pattern over a period of weeks.
B- Increasing frequency of capillary blood glucose testing to avoid hypo- and hyperglycaemia, as these may exacerbate stress and can affect performance. Remember that insulin requirements can drop quite sharply after the stressful period is over and reduced basal patterns may be needed.

3- Psychological support

4- Benefits of relaxation skills and exercise in reducing stress are well known. Exercise gives them a feeling of well-being and may relieve symptoms of stress.

Most stressful situations are unpredicted in children. One of the essential aspects of pump therapy is to know how to handle unanticipated stressful situations. The main feature to manage these situations is careful monitoring, reviewing and adjusting.

5.8 Puberty and menstruation

Puberty is a difficult time for children, especially ones with type 1 diabetes, due to hormonal, psychological, body and environmental changes. This is a period when insulin requirements change in a manner that is difficult to predict. It requires discussion with your patients to avoid frustration and will require close supervision for adjustments to achieve stable control.

Often insulin requirements increase during puberty. Insulin's effectiveness declines by about 30% to 50% because growth and sexual hormones create insulin resistance.

The premenstrual period in girls with type 1 diabetes may lead to hyperglycaemia and increased insulin requirements. Many report their blood sugar tends to increase 3 to 5 days prior to the beginning of their period. They may require a different basal profile or may be managed with temporary basal rates. Their blood sugar then returns to normal within the first few days after their period has started.

5.9 Coffee and alcohol

Coffee: Although most children don't drink coffee, we need to make teenagers aware of the effect of caffeine on blood glucose control. Coffee may have carbohydrate content due to the presence of milk. Coffee can also cause a degree of insulin resistance so that a larger amount of insulin may be needed as a temporary basal rate or bolus with food. This varies from person to person. This is also applicable to other caffeinated drinks, such as cola/energy drinks etc.

Alcohol: Alcohol can affect blood glucose levels, so it is important to explain this to your patients and their parents/carers. This can help them to stay safe. Alcohol can have a large impact on glucose levels. It prevents the release of glucose from the liver (hepatic gluconeogenesis) in the fasting state and increases the risk of hypoglycaemia, especially overnight. It is recommended that a snack containing carbohydrate should be taken without a bolus to slow alcohol absorption and prevent hypoglycaemia. Alternatively, a temporary basal rate may be used after alcohol to reduce the insulin effect, particularly in the liver. At the same time, the high sugar content in alcoholic beverages may cause a rise in glucose while drinking.

Learning and refining from experience is the best way to determine how to manage glucose, which will respond differently to different beverage type and quantity. It is advisable to use no or smaller bolus initially (reduce ICR by half), monitor frequently, set alarms to wake up to test and to inform others of the risk of going low and what to do if this happens.

5.10 Steroids

Steroids, such as prednisolone, hydrocortisone and dexamethasone are commonly used in children for inflammatory and autoimmune conditions (e.g. asthma, eczema, croup and inflammatory bowel disease) and may also be used in chronic diseases such as nephritic syndrome and rheumatoid arthritis. High doses of steroids cause insulin resistance and will increase insulin requirements dramatically. This may be termed steroid induced hyperglycaemia. This will warrant temporary, additional and more active glycaemic management. Severity of hyperglycaemia will depend on type, time and duration of steroid course.

This can be tackled by:
1. Consider increasing monitoring. A close recording (4–6 hourly) of blood glucose should be kept to work out individual requirements.
2. An increase in basal of 30–50% initially may be needed during times of maximal hyperglycaemia. Increases of up to 200–300% are not uncommon.
3. Consider changing ICR.
4. During steroid weaning or cessation, insulin requirements can drop back very quickly and close monitoring of blood sugar and adjustments are needed.
5. Refresh diabetes education with patient

5.11 Psychological aspects of insulin pump therapy

Some patients have reported downsides to pump therapy that affect children's quality of life. These include the constant reminder of the diseased state, constant attachment to the pump, visibility of the device, concerns about breakdown and reliance on the device. Psychological factors are the main challenges of pump therapy, besides remembering to bolus.

These are some useful points to consider for children on a pump:
1- Given the complexity of diabetes management, children on insulin pump are likely to benefit from a multidisciplinary team of practitioners who are knowledgeable about and experienced in the specific challenges at this age.
2- Children interested in pump therapy may need to be scheduled to meet with your team psychologist to further assess behavioral aspects of pump readiness and to discuss the psychosocial adjustment to this form of insulin treatment.
3- Psychological assessment and support advice for children with diabetes, especially when starting on the insulin pump and regularly afterwards, as and when needed.
4- Allow sufficient time for insulin pump training (not to be undertaken when rushed or under pressure). This reduces the sense of threat and provides the family and their child with a sense of control in a more relaxed setting.
5- Keep the 'emotional temperature' whilst changing as calm as possible to prevent the development of negative associations.
6- Parents need to avoid overprotectiveness as this can stifle natural drives toward independence in an older child. This can also give rise to oppositional behaviour (food refusal, lack of cooperation over routines, etc.). Remember that noncompliance with the task of carbohydrate counting may be used as a weapon against parents if a child is angry.
7- A child's feelings to their insulin pump will often 'mirror' their parent's feelings toward the pump.

8- Having reasonable expectations is very important (not setting the standard too high as to be consistently unattainable and thus demotivating).
9- When parental anxieties about a child's diabetes can be contained (remaining outwardly calm), it can prevent the spread of apprehension/fearfulness in their child (feelings are contagious).
10- Avoid frequent critical or negative reactions to poor blood sugar control as it can damage self-esteem, reduce motivation and encourage rebellious attitudes.
11- Try to focus on behaviours rather than outcomes as this is more productive (as the former is more directly under the control of your patient), with affirmation / praise given for any positive efforts to control blood sugar.

6 Appendices

Appendix I: Infection prevention
Appendix II: Fasting record sheet
Appendix III: Travel checklist
Appendix IV: Blood glucose conversion chart

Appendix I: Infection prevention

Signs and symptoms of infection

a- Local
- 1- Redness or warm area
- 2- Drainage (clear, cloudy, white, yellow or bloody)
- 3- Unpleasant odour
- 4- Pain or discomfort at the site

b- Systemic
- 1- Fever or chills
- 2- Nausea or vomiting
- 3- Unexplained hyperglycaemia

How to prevent skin problems and infections

1. Wash your hands thoroughly with water and antibacterial soap before and after handling pump, pump supplies, site dressings and medications.
2. Inspect your site twice daily, once in the morning and once in the evening. Look for signs of infection (mentioned earlier).
3. When preparing your site, use an antibacterial soap solution. Cleanse the skin in a circular motion, from the inside to the outside. A skin protectant such as Skin Prep® may be applied if needed. A 7.0 cm diameter area is best. Allow your skin to dry naturally.
4. Ensure contents of sterile package have not been opened or damaged. If the integrity of the package has been breached, discard and use a new one.
5. Antibiotic (local/systemic) treatment may be needed. Patients/parents may need to consult their healthcare provider if they are having problems with skin irritation or infection.
6. Never recap used needles.

Appendix II: Fasting record sheet

Use a chart to record your patient's blood glucose while they are fasting, then re-assess their basal rate. They may find it helpful to mark the boxes with a tick (✓) where you are planning to test blood glucose (for some you may elect to stop earlier than midday).

Morning and early afternoon testing: early breakfast, start blood testing from 10 am – 6 pm, miss lunch.

TIME (HRS)	07:00	08:00	09:00	10:00	11:00	12:00	13:00	14:00	15:00	16:00	17:00	18:00
FASTING (water only)												
BGL	✓		✓		✓		✓		✓		✓	

BGL = Blood glucose level

Afternoon/evening test: no eating from midday until 10 pm, state time of last meal and last injection/bolus.

TIME (HRS)	12:00	13:00	14:00	15:00	16:00	17:00	18:00	19:00	20:00	21:00	22:00	23:00
FASTING (water only)												
BGL	✓		✓		✓		✓		✓		✓	

Overnight and morning testing: your patient should not eat from 8 pm until midday the next day (finish earlier if needed) they should miss breakfast. Document the time of the last meal and last bolus.

TIME (HRS)	MIDNIGHT	01:00	02:00	03:00	04:00	05:00	06:00	07:00	08:00	09:00	10:00
FASTING (water only)											
BGL	✓			✓			✓		✓		✓

Appendix III- Travel checklist

1- A back-up vacation loaner pump
2- Infusion sets and cartridges
3- Insulin (rapid and long-acting)
4- Blood glucose monitor and test strips
5- Skin preparation dressings or adhesive
6- A list of current pump settings
7- Extra pump clip and/or pump case
8- Extra battery cap and cartridge cap for pump
9- Lancing device and lancets
10- Extra batteries for pump/meter
11- Syringes or insulin pens
12- Sharps container
13- Ketone test strips
14- Hypoglycaemia treatment (glucose tabs, glucagon, etc.)
15- Any other medications you require
16- Copies of all prescriptions
17- Copies of physician's orders for dosing of rapid and long-acting insulin
18- Emergency contact numbers

Appendix IV: management of hyperglycaemia in a patient on insulin pump

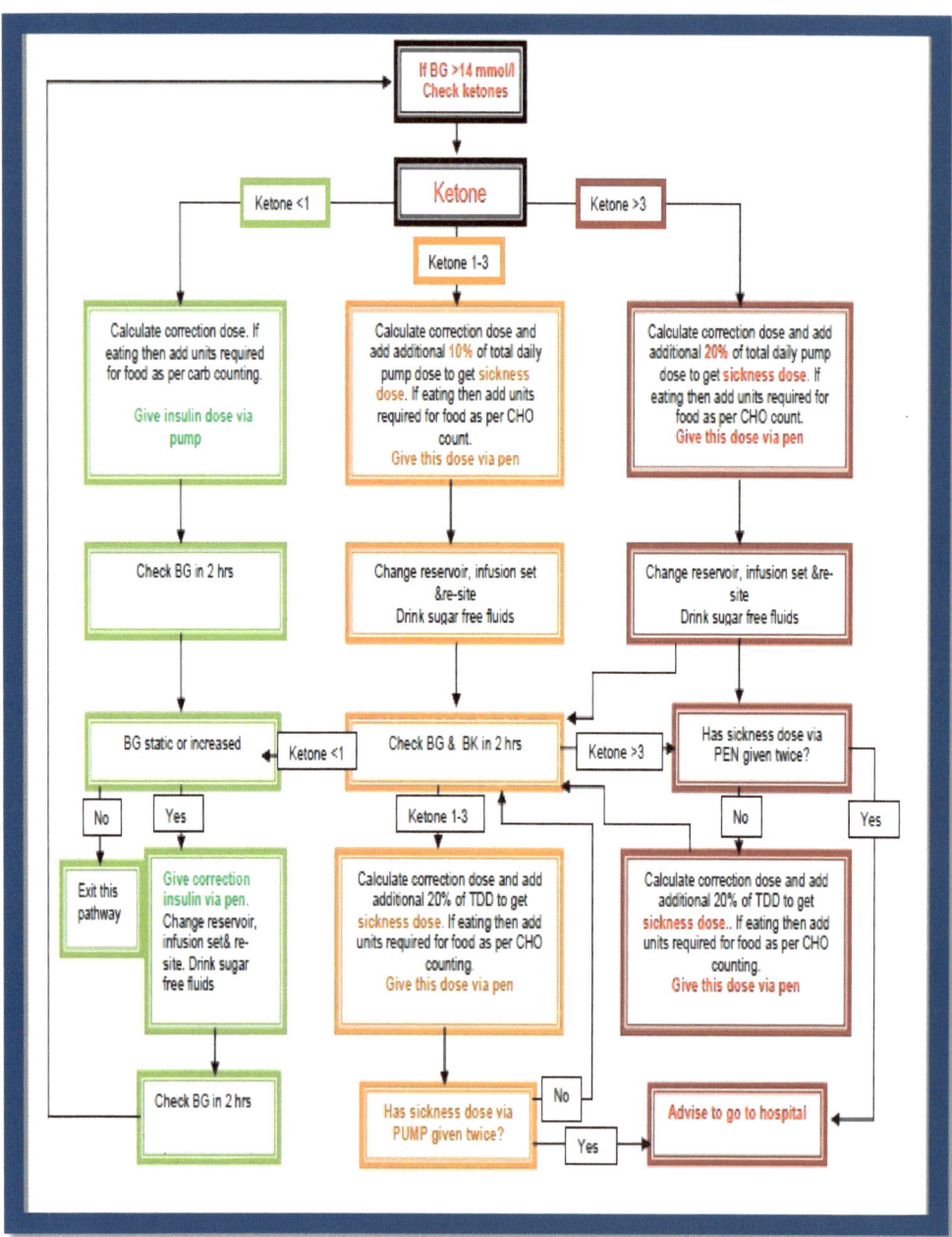

Appendix V: Blood Glucose Conversion Chart (mmol/L - mg/dl)

Mmol	Mg	Mmol	Mg	Mmol	Mg	Mmol	Mg	Mmol	Mg
2.0	36	6.0	108	10.0	180	14.0	252	18.0	324
2.1	38	6.1	110	10.1	182	14.1	254	18.1	326
2.2	39	6.2	112	10.2	184	14.2	256	18.2	328
2.3	41	6.3	113	10.3	185	14.3	257	18.3	329
2.4	43	6.4	115	10.4	187	14.4	259	18.4	331
2.5	45	6.5	117	10.5	189	14.5	261	18.5	333
2.6	47	6.6	119	10.6	191	14.6	263	18.6	335
2.7	48	6.7	121	10.7	193	14.7	265	18.7	337
2.8	50	6.8	122	10.8	194	14.8	266	18.8	338
2.9	52	6.9	124	10.9	196	14.9	268	18.9	340
3.0	54	7.0	126	11.0	198	15.0	270	19.0	342
3.1	56	7.1	128	11.1	200	15.1	272	19.1	344
3.2	58	7.2	130	11.2	202	15.2	274	19.2	346
3.3	59	7.3	131	11.3	203	15.3	275	19.3	347
3.4	61	7.4	133	11.4	205	15.4	277	19.4	349
3.5	63	7.5	135	11.5	207	15.5	279	19.5	351
3.6	64	7.6	137	11.6	209	15.6	281	19.6	353
3.7	66	7.7	139	11.7	211	15.7	283	19.7	355
3.8	68	7.8	140	11.8	212	15.8	284	19.8	356
3.9	70	7.9	142	11.9	214	15.9	286	19.9	358
4.0	72	8.0	144	12.0	216	16.0	288	20.0	360
4.1	74	8.1	146	12.1	218	16.1	290	20.1	362
4.2	76	8.2	148	12.2	220	16.2	292	20.2	364
4.3	77	8.3	149	12.3	221	16.3	293	20.3	365
4.4	79	8.4	151	12.4	223	16.4	295	20.4	367
4.5	81	8.5	153	12.5	225	16.5	297	20.5	369
4.6	83	8.6	155	12.6	227	16.6	299	20.6	371
4.7	85	8.7	157	12.7	229	16.7	301	20.7	373
4.8	86	8.8	158	12.8	230	16.8	302	20.8	374
4.9	88	8.9	160	12.9	232	16.9	304	20.9	376
5.0	90	9.0	162	13.0	234	17.0	306	21.0	378
5.1	92	9.1	164	13.1	236	17.1	308	21.1	380
5.2	94	9.2	166	13.2	238	17.2	310	21.2	382
5.3	95	9.3	167	13.3	239	17.3	311	21.3	383
5.4	97	9.4	169	13.4	241	17.4	313	21.4	385
5.5	99	9.5	171	13.5	243	17.5	315	21.5	387
5.6	100	9.6	172	13.6	245	17.6	317	21.6	388
5.7	102	9.7	174	13.7	247	17.7	319	21.7	390
5.8	104	9.8	176	13.8	248	17.8	320	21.8	392
5.9	106	9.9	178	13.9	250	17.9	322	21.9	394

Index:

Adjusting insulin to carbohydrate ratio, 56
Advantages of pumps, 5
Alarm Feature, 65
Alcohol, ii, 71, 90, 105
Basal rate calculation, 25
Before you start, 17
Benefits of insulin pump therapy, 4
beta cells, 2
Blood glucose targets, 33
Bolus options, 85
Calculating ICR, 30
Cannula, 3, 6, 9, 11, 12, 14, 17, 19, 20, 21, 22, 23, 37, 38, 47, 48, 49, 58, 64, 96, 97
Coffee, ii, 90, 105
Continuous glucose monitoring (CGM), i, 56, 59, 65
Continuous subcutaneous insulin infusion', 2, 4
Correction Bolus Formula, 32
Correction dose calculation, 32
Cost of pumps, 8
CSII, 2, 4, 17
Daily overlay view, 70
Daily summaries, 71
Dawn effect, 75
Dawn phenomenon, 57
Decision making, 68
Diabetic ketoacidosis, i, iv, 39, 51
Disadvantages of pumps, 5
DKA, 51
Dual wave, 86
Dusk phenomenon, 58
Emergency kit, 36
Emergency surgery, 100
Exercise, ii, i, 4, 8, 12, 13, 15, 21, 32, 36, 37, 38, 42, 43, 44, 46, 52, 53, 61, 62, 63, 68, 71, 72, 73, 75, 82, 87, 90, 92, 93, 94, 95, 96, 97
Fast-acting insulin, 4, 17, 24, 25, 32, 35, 42, 43, 51, 78
Fasting, ii, 53, 55, 71, 82, 83, 90, 102, 103, 105, 110
Fat, 83
Fibre, 83
Follow-up, i, 16, 24, 25, 36, 37
Food, ii, 2, 4, 6, 12, 13, 17, 30, 31, 32, 35, 40, 42, 43, 45, 47, 51, 53, 54, 55, 56, 66, 68, 71, 72, 75, 77, 78, 79, 80, 81, 82, 83, 84, 85, 88, 91, 102, 105, 106
Glycaemic index, 78
Glycaemic variability, 74
Goals and expectations, 14
HbA_{1c}, i, 1, 7, 8, 10, 12, 13, 17, 25, 29, 37, 63, 65, 75
Holidays, ii, 90, 100
Hormones, 46
Hospital admission, ii, 90, 98
Hyperglycaemia, 46
Hypoglycaemia, 40
Hypoglycaemia prevention, 42
Hypoglycaemia unawareness, 74
Illness, i, 4, 6, 10, 18, 31, 32, 36, 39, 46, 49, 51, 52, 53, 82, 90, 97, 100, 103
Illness, 90
Indications, 17
Infection, ii, 46, 49, 108, 109
Infusion site management, 11
Injection sites, 11
Insulin on Board (IOB), 88
Insulin on-board (IOB), 33
Insulin pump basics, 11
Insulin to carbohydrate ratio, 30
Interstitial fluid, 62
Islets of Langerhans, 2
Ketones, i, 12, 39, 46, 50, 51, 52, 93, 95, 98, 99, 100
Limitations of pumps, 6
Mean absolute difference, 70
Menstruation, ii, 90, 104
Metal / steel cannula, 20
Multiwave, 86
Negative correction, 44
Outliers, 73
Pancreas, 2, 4, 7, 67, 68
Patch pump, 8, 9, 10
Pattern, 72
Post-operative care, 100
Protein, 83, 84, 85, 87
Psychological aspects, ii, 90, 106
Puberty, ii, 90, 104
Pump accessories, 19
Pump choices, 8
Ramadan, ii, 53, 90, 102
Real time, 61
Reservoirs, 21
Retrospective analysis, 61
School, ii, 90, 91
Selection criteria, 17
Sensor augmented pump, 7
Showering, 13, 14, 21, 92
Sites for cannula, 22

Sleeping, 92
Social Life, 90
Square or extended wave, 85
Steroids, ii, 47, 90, 105
Stress, 46, 103
Surgeries, ii, 90, 98
Swimming, 6, 13, 14, 21, 35, 75, 92, 94, 97
Symptoms of hypoglycaemia, 41
Technical issues/failure, 35
Temporary basal rates, i, 16, 36
Testing and adjusting basal rate, 52
Tethered pump, 8
Time zones, 101
Transition, 23
Travel, ii, 90, 100, 101, 103
Trend, 59, 65, 66, 67, 72
Tubing and cannula, 3
Unplanned situations, ii, 90, 103
Uses of insulin pump, 8